ULCER AND NON-ULCER DYSPEPSIAS

PRACTICAL CLINICAL MEDICINE

Series Editors J. Fry and G. Sandler

ULCER AND NON-ULCER DYSPEPSIAS

Edited by
M. Lancaster-Smith

Consultant Gastroenterologist
Queen Mary's Hospital
Sidcup
Kent

WKAP ARCHIEF

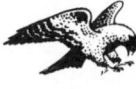
MTP PRESS LIMITED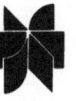
a member of the KLUWER ACADEMIC PUBLISHERS GROUP
LANCASTER / BOSTON / THE HAGUE / DORDRECHT

Published in the UK and Europe by
MTP Press Limited
Falcon House
Lancaster, England

British Library Cataloguing in Publication Data

Ulcer and non-ulcer dyspepsias.—(Practical
clinical medicine)
1. Peptic ulcer
I. Lancaster-Smith, Michael   II. Series
616.3′43   RC821

ISBN-13: 978-0-85200-691-7   e-ISBN-13: 978-94-010-9928-8
DOI: 10.1007/978-94-010-9928-8

Published in the USA by
MTP Press
A division of Kluwer Academic Publishers
101 Philip Drive
Norwell, MA 02061, USA

Library of Congress Cataloging in Publication Data
Ulcer and non-ulcer dyspepsias.

(Practical clinical medicine)
Includes bibliographies and index.
1. Peptic ulcer.   2. Dyspepsia.
I. Lancaster-Smith, Michael   II. Series
[DNLM: 1 Dispepsia—physiopathology.   2. Peptic
Ulcer—physiopathology.   WI 350 U36]
RC821.U43   1986   616.3′43   86–27521

ISBN-13: 978-0-85200-691-7

Contents

List of Contributors

Dr M. J. G. Farthing
Senior Lecturer
Department of
Gastroenterology
St Bartholomew's Hospital
London EC1A 7BE

Prof M. Hobsley
The Middlesex Hospital
London W1N 8AA

Dr J. G. C. Kingham
Consultant Physician
Morriston Hospital
Swansea, Wales

Dr M. Lancaster-Smith
Consultant
Gastroenterologist
Queen Mary's Hospital
Sidcup, Kent

Dr A. J. M. Watson
Research Fellow
Department of
Gastroenterology
St Bartholomew's Hospital
London EC1A 7BE

Dr P. F. Whitfield
The Middlesex Hospital
London W1N 8AA

Series Editors' Foreword

Backing up the pioneering medical researchers and experimenters are the phalanxes and cohorts of practising clinicians in district general hospitals and in general practice who may have to implement and apply any breakthroughs and advances in practical and realistic terms. This they cannot, and should not, be expected to do without careful consideration and analysis. It is essential, therefore, to have regular reviews of the growing points of medicine which are constructively critical as well as being enthusiastic and which can present the issues and implications clearly and fairly to clinicians.

The *Practical Clinical Medicine* series is designed to provide such regular reviews on selected subjects. Each volume is under the charge of an invited editor who selects his team of 4–6 experts. Each contribution is an authoritative, detailed and referenced examination of his topic, is clearly presented in an understandable manner and is practical, relevant and applicable to everyday clinical practice.

The series is intended as a means of communication between researchers and practising clinicians. It is dedicated to generalists who provide primary health care in general practice and to generalists providing secondary medical care in district general hospitals. Both are involved in applying good general practical clinical medicine for their patients, but can only succeed in a climate of constant review and examination.

JOHN FRY
GERALD SANDLER

Introduction

The disorders discussed in this volume are undoubtedly amongst the commonest reasons for seeking medical opinion and advice. Peptic inflammation and ulceration of the oesophagus, stomach and duodenum constitute approximately 50% of referrals from general practitioners to hospital gastroenterology clinics in the United Kingdom. In addition nonulcer dyspepsia in which category it is now customary to include the irritable bowel syndrome account for a further 40% of referred patients.

The epidemiological profile of peptic ulcer has changed significantly during this century and re-evaluation of this information may hopefully provide clues to the aetiology of gastric and duodenal ulceration. Furthermore during the past decade technological advances have encouraged vigorous research into the pathophysiological mechanisms involved in gastro-oesophageal reflux, peptic ulcer and non-ulcer dyspepsia.

The advent of highly effective drugs that heal peptic lesions and the coincident burgeoning of upper gastrointestinal endoscopy have stimulated numerous long-term studies of these disorders. Their behaviour is now clearly understood and their recurrent nature has been unequivocally confirmed. The widespread use of endoscopy has shown that many patients with symptoms suggestive of peptic disease have no mucosal abnormality in the upper gastrointestinal tract. Rather it seems that many of them have functional disturbances of the small or large intestine which are now being more accurately defined.

Surgery for all forms of peptic disease has declined during the past decade but this trend is perhaps reversing in duodenal ulcer management due to the generally favourable result that the majority of patients experience after proximal gastric vagotomy.

It is not the intention of this book to comprehensively cover the total field of peptic disease and non-ulcer dyspepsias but rather to review those areas and topics which are likely to be of special interest to general practitioners.

M. LANCASTER-SMITH

1

PATHOPHYSIOLOGY OF PEPTIC ULCER

M. HOBSLEY and P. F. WHITFIELD

INTRODUCTORY CONCEPTS

Definition

Although clinicians think they know what they mean when they use the term peptic ulcer, a precise and concise definition is not easy to achieve. The fundamental concept is that the ulcer is related to the proteolytic action of the mixture of hydrochloric acid and pepsin secreted by the parietal and chief cells of the stomach. It follows that the diagnosis can only be entertained in those patients in which these cells function (as summarized in Schwartz's famous dictum 'no acid, no ulcer'), and in geographical sites to which the acid/pepsin mixture has access.

The Necessity for Acid/Pepsin

The necessity for acid/pepsin rules out the possibility of a peptic ulcer in patients with complete ('histamine-fast') achlor-

1

hydria, and in patients with inflammation and ulceration of the oesophagus after total gastrectomy ('alkaline oesophagitis'). Along the same lines – and despite the fact that this point is rarely made by those writing on the subject – it is most unlikely that the shallow multiple ulcers occurring in the stomach and duodenum of very ill, shocked patients can owe much to acid/pepsin secretion for their origin[1]. The reduced tissue perfusion of shock turns off the secretion of acid/pepsin by the stomach like a tap, and evidence has recently been obtained, notably by T. K. Hunt in California, and Fiddian-Green in Boston, that the so-called 'stress ulceration' is due to tissue necrosis resulting from the low tissue oxygen tension produced by inadequate blood flow.

Site of Ulcers

Of great interest, and surely a fact of great importance for understanding the pathophysiology of peptic ulceration, is the fact that peptic ulcers never seem to occur in acid/pepsin secreting tissue[2,3]. The commonest peptic ulcer these days is the duodenal. The second commonest is the stomach, but the ulcers do not seem to be situated in the corporeal or acid-secreting mucosa, but in the antral mucosa which contains no parietal or chief cells and secretes an alkaline mucus. While this statement is obviously true of the commoner pre-pyloric and incisural ulcers, it also seems to be true of the higher ulcers: even when these occur near the oesophageal hiatus; they seem to be sited in a tongue of antral mucosa that extends upwards from the anatomical antrum along the lesser curvature of the stomach. Another example of this general rule is the anastomotic ulcer that may occur in the vicinity of the stoma of a gastrojejunostomy or a Bilroth II type of partial gastrectomy. In both these operations, there is a direct connection between stomach or stomach-remnant on the one hand, and the jejunum on the other. If the surgical procedure has failed to reduce gastric secretion sufficiently, ulceration ensues: apart from unusual cases in which the ulceration occurs on the gastric side of the anastomosis because of local factors such as the surgical use of non-absorbable sutures, this ulceration is confined to the jejunal side of the junction. Finally, when there is an ectopic site of functioning parietal mucosa, e.g. in a Meckel's diverticulum, any peptic ulcer that results again arises in the ileal mucosa at the boundary of the island of heterotopic gastric tissue. In other words, the tissues that secrete the acid/pepsin mixture seem to possess infinite resistance to the digestive activity of what they secrete.

Histopathology

To naked-eye inspection, a typical peptic ulcer is circular in outline and has vertical walls: hence the textbook description that it is punched-out (Figure 1.1a and b). This tendency for the walls to be vertical is noticeable on histological examination, which also reveals that, at least in a 'chronic' ulcer, the destruction proceeds deeply into the muscular layer and indeed often through it, so that the floor of the ulcer (if free perforation has not occurred) is only fibrous tissue or else a neighbouring organ such as the liver.

The use above of the term 'chronic' ulcer reminds us to comment on the use of that term, and of its antithesis, 'acute'. The description 'acute peptic ulcer' has been used, confusingly, to describe two different entities – the shallow erosions in shocked patients and the punched-out lesions that can be seen in patients in whom the history of indigestion seems to be very short. Certainly erosions or stress ulcers are better terms for the first entity. With regard to the second, surgeons used to be taught that whether the ulcer had been present for a short or a long time might affect whether, when operating for a perforated duodenal ulcer, one should consider adding a procedure for reducing gastric secretion, in an attempt at curing the ulcer diathesis, to the standard procedure for sealing the perforation. It was said that one could distinguish a chronic

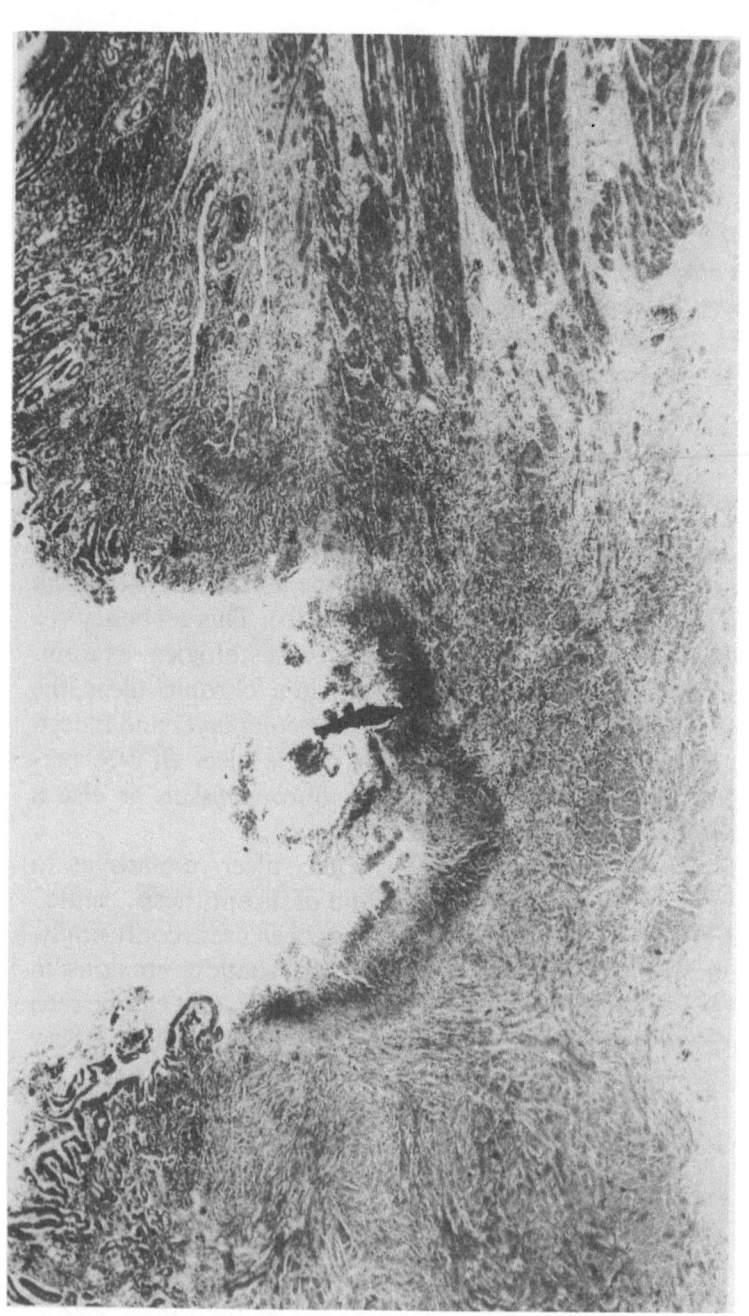

Figure 1.1a Photomicrograph of a small chronic gastric ulcer. The walls are vertical and the ulcer has punched partway through the muscle. × 15

from an acute ulcer not only from the history, but also from the amount of fibrosis found at operation around the ulcer. This does not seem to have proved a useful concept, since there is often a marked lack of correlation between history and operative findings. It is probably best to drop the distinction between acute and chronic.

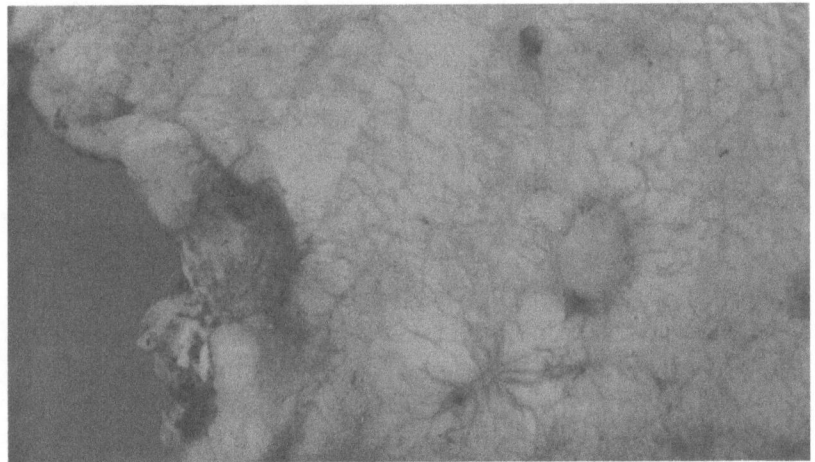

Figure 1.1b Post-operative specimen of a gastric ulcer showing the circular punched-out appearance with near-vertical walls

Combining the results reviewed under the headings of site and histopathology, we may define peptic ulcer disease as vertical walled ulceration affecting the gastrointestinal tract near acid/pepsin secreting epithelium.

Trauma

There are two aspects to the aetiology of an ulcer: what produces the breach in the epithelium; and what prevents the ulcer from healing?

It must be said that there is no firm evidence about the first aspect, but the traditional view is that trauma is implicated.

In the case of gastric ulcers, it is pointed out that the common site is somewhere along the lesser curvature, i.e., in the 'Magenstrasse' of the German descriptions, the channel that represents the shortest route for boluses of food to take from oesophagus to duodenum, and therefore the area that might be expected to sustain most frictional trauma. For duodenal ulcer, the suggestion is that a mixture of food solution with acid/pepsin passes through the pylorus, when the latter relaxes, in a forceful jet resulting from the propulsive contractions of the antral muscles: this jet strikes the wall of the duodenum somewhere in its first part, and so determines the common site of a duodenal ulcer.

Against the hypothesis of trauma is the fact that traumatic ulcers in skin have a very different histological appearance. Even if a traumatic ulcer in skin has vertical walls at its inception, the process of healing rapidly results in the walls becoming terraced and inclined gently towards the middle of the ulcer. This difference does not rule out trauma as the primary factor: the orientation of the walls may be a function of columnar epithelium in the stomach and duodenum as distinct from the stratified squamous epithelium of skin. This possibility may help to explain the phenomenon known as Barrett's ulcer: when excessive reflux of acid/pepsin and bile from the stomach into the lower oesophagus produces oesophagitis, typical peptic ulceration of the oesophagus only occurs if long-standing reflux has given rise to a metaplastic change in the mucosa lining the lower oesophagus, from squamous to columnar. Nevertheless, one must repeat that there is virtually no evidence in direct support of trauma as the initiating factor.

AETIOLOGY

Peptic ulcer disease is usually considered to be a consequence of an imbalance of the 'aggressive' action of gastric acid and pepsin and the mucosal defences. Gastric acid and pepsin are treated as a single entity, since in man at least, a change in one is usually associated with a change in the other. With this model in mind, an increase in acid/pepsin, or a decrease in mucosal resistance beyond some unknown threshold would result in ulceration, whilst a change of both factors in the same direction would not necessarily produce an ulcer. The successful treatment of peptic ulcer should therefore be the reversal of the imbalance.

Aggressive Factors

Excess Acid/Pepsin

From the idea that acid was necessary to produce a peptic ulcer, it seemed a small step to postulate that excess acid was the root cause of peptic ulceration. When the augmented histamine test was developed[4], so that acid secretion could reliably be maximally stimulated and collected from the stomach without contamination with food, this postulate seemed to be confirmed, at least for duodenal ulcer. It was true that there seemed to be no evidence of an increased ability to secrete acid in patients with gastric ulcer. However, there seemed to be no doubt about a strong association between raised secretion and duodenal ulcer – mean values for maximal secretion in groups of duodenal ulcer patients were 50–100% higher than those in control groups[5]. Nevertheless, even in duodenal ulcer patients, there was considerable overlap: while there were patients with duodenal ulcer with maximal gastric secretion rates well above the normal limits, and control subjects with rates below the lower limit of the duodenal ulcer group, the majority of duodenal ulcer patients have maximal secretion rates within the normal range.

Considerable effort has been spent on exploring the possibility that at least part of the overlap was due to errors of collection (swallowed saliva, sequestration of acid between gastric mucosal folds, pyloric losses and duodenogastric reflux)[6] or due to differences in secretion-related factors (stature, age, sex)[7]. However, to date the middle ground of overlap stubbornly persists despite all such efforts.

Gastric secretion is a function of height and age. In the range 150–200 cm, maximal gastric secretion increases linearly with height. Age has a negative effect, but is not as marked as height. Even taking these factors into account, and with the eradication of the commonly found sex difference in gastric secretion, the duodenal ulcer patients still secrete significantly more than controls. There may be major ethnic factors too, since Scottish duodenal ulcer patients have significantly higher màximal acid òutput than do Chinese patients even after such factors as weight, blood group, and family history are taken into account[8].

A more recent finding has been of the effect of chronic cigarette smoking. Many studies have been carried out on the effect of acute cigarette smoking, but the results are inconclusive. This may be due to differing doses of nicotine between the studies, or the failure to allow for such factors as pyloric loss and duodeno-gastric reflux on the acid secretion. Whatever the reasons, the probable effect of acute smoking is small, whilst recent research has uncovered a considerable effect of chronic smoking. In one study[9], both acute and chronic smoking were studied in duodenal ulcer patients, and chronic smoking was studied in patients with non-ulcer dyspepsia. The smoking of four cigarettes in 40 minutes did not influence basal gastric secretion of acid or pepsin, or serum pepsinogen I and gastrin concentrations. However, in both patient groups, pentagastrin-stimulated acid secretion and fasting serum pepsinogen I concentrations were significantly higher among habitual heavy smokers than among non-smokers. In a second report[10], the histamine-stimulated maximal acid volume in duodenal ulcer patients, corrected for pyloric loss and duodenogastric reflux, was statistically significantly correlated with an index of the total number of cigarettes smoked. That is, the more cigarettes the patient had smoked, the greater their maximal gastric secretion. This increase seems to occur in healthy controls, but nevertheless, chronic smoking appears to be another factor influencing gastric secretion. Duodenal ulcer disease is principally found in males, with an age of onset commonly in their thirties. Cigarette smoking may be found to have an important bearing on this sex and age distribution, and also on the epidemiological pattern of the disease in this century. High maximal gastric secretion is associated with large parietal cell mass, and therefore chronic smoking would be expected somehow to increase this cell mass. Chronic sham feeding of dogs for six weeks produced a 27% increase in maximal acid output, an effect that was reversed after cessation of sham feeding. Since no effect was seen in denervated dogs, it was concluded that vagal stimulation led to a higher parietal cell mass. The major trophic hormone for the stomach is gastrin, and abnormal gastrin secretion can lead to very high acid secretion, and eventually duodenal ulcer (the Zollinger–Ellison syndrome). Further, it has been shown that, in rats, chronic administration of nicotine increases maximal acid output. There remains to be discovered the route by which chronic smoking leads to increased gastric secretion. An increased vagal drive, if it exists, is thought to account for the greater sensitivity of duodenal ulcer patients to both endogenous and exogenous gastrin. Increased hormonal stimulation may also be responsible, but in most duodenal ulcer patients the fasting gastrin concentrations are normal.

Enough Acid/Pepsin

It is salutary to approach the problem from the opposite direction. If too much acid is not essential patients may develop a duodenal ulcer despite having an acid production in the normal range; but if (and this seems to remain true) no acid is synonymous with no ulcer, then what is the minimal secretory ability that can permit a duodenal ulcer to exist? There is evidence from two sources. One is the lower secretory limit of large groups of duodenal ulcer patients. The other is the secretion rates of patients who do or do not develop recurrent peptic ulceration after operations such as partial gastrectomy or vagotomy that are designed to reduce gastric secretion. With regard to maximally-stimulated secretion, and using the measurement of Vg (gastric secretion in millilitres per hour, corrected for pyloric loss and duodeno-gastric reflux), the values appear to be 100 and 140 respectively. These are approximately equivalent to a maximal gastric acid output of 8.7 mmol/h and 11.89 mmol/h. If the acid-reducing operation was vagotomy, then insulin-stimulated secretion after operation must not differ from basal secretion, i.e. the vagotomy must be complete. If a subject is found, under the respective conditions detailed, to secrete less acid than the appropriate threshold, then the chance that he has a duodenal ulcer is less than 2.5%.

The Acid/Alkali Gradient and Ulcer Location

If a small quantity of acid can produce an ulcer in some people but not in others, then an obvious possibility is that resistance to the digestive properties of acid/pepsin might vary from one individual to another. This concept is developed in greater detail in the subsequent sections, but one aspect in particular is considered here. The natural antidote to acid is alkali, and the natural direction for liquids to flow in the alimentary tract is caudad. Acid produced in the stomach passes into the duodenum and is there neutralized by bicarbonate from the duodenum, the gall bladder and the pancreas. The more acid is produced in the stomach, the further will it penetrate along the duodenum before it can be neutralized. On the other hand, if the stomach makes relatively little acid, then neutralization will be complete even in the antrum, perhaps with the aid of a little reflux of duodenal bicarbonate back into the stomach. It is fascinating to note that the tendency to hypersecretion of acid in patients with a duodenal ulcer is not paralleled in patients with gastric ulcer. Indeed, in the latter group a higher secretion in the pre-pyloric ulcers, a normal secretion in those

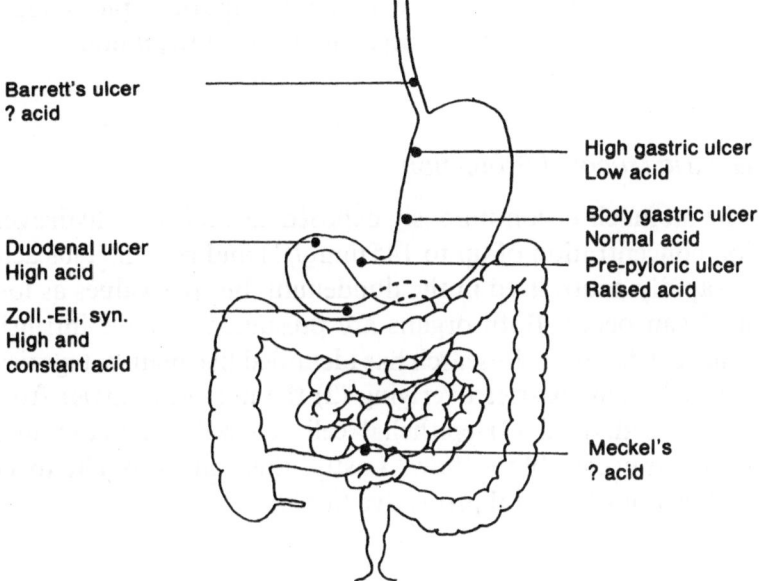

Figure 1.2 Peptic ulcer and maximal gastric acid secretion

with ulcers at the incisura, and a low secretion in those with ulcers high on the lesser curvature demonstrate this gradient (Figure 1.2). So does the tendency for the gross hypersecretion of acid in patients with the Zollinger–Ellison syndrome to be associated with ulcers at more distal sites in the small intestine than usual, in the second or third parts of the duodenum, or even in the jejunum.

Protective Factors in Peptic Ulcer Disease

Over the past decade, the mucosal defences have received increasing research attention, mainly in animals, and the first part of this section examines the fruits of this labour and the implications for the attack/defence model of peptic ulceration. Most work has been done on the stomach, presumably because of its accessibility and the greater knowledge of its physiology, even though most human ulcers are in the duodenum.

Gastric Mucosal Protection

The stomach is continuously exposed to acid (of a hydrogen ion concentration of up to 145 mmol/1) and pepsin. This acid is rapidly neutralized in the duodenum, but pH values as low as 2 can occur. Both organs are presumed to have intrinsic mucosal defences. Research has identified five main categories: (1) the mucus barrier overlying (2) the mucosal barrier from which is derived (3) epithelial cell renewal, all maintained by (4) mucosal blood flow. Lastly, there are thought to be endogenous humoral protective factors.

The Mucus Barrier

Gastroduodenal mucus is constantly secreted by surface epithelial cells as a glycoprotein-rich, viscous, elastic, water-insoluble gel (but itself 95% water) adherent to the mucosal surface. The protective function consists of acting as a stable mixing barrier (together with HCO_3 secretion) to luminal acid, a diffusion barrier to pepsin, and together with soluble mucus, as a lubricant. The thickness of the adherent mucus is variable, but can be up to one millimetre. It is a remarkably tough barrier, since the thickness, in the short term in the rat, is essentially unchanged after such insults as 100% ethanol, 80 mmol/1 sodium taurocholate, indomethacin 30 mg/kg, 0.6 mol/1 HCl or 2 mol/1 NaCl[11]. The mucus barrier is, however, readily permeable to ions and small molecules. The penetration of hydrogen ions is thought to be curtailed by the active secretion of HCO_3 by antral and fundic mucosa, which becomes trapped in the mucus and creates a pH gradient (pH 7 at the mucosal surface)[12]. Presumably, pepsin would also be inactive at this pH. Aspirin and bile salts impair the maintenance of this pH gradient. This role for a portion of the non-parietal component of gastric juice has only recently been acknowledged, and its contribution to the protection of the epithelium is not known. The amount of bicarbonate secreted is small (about 400–500 μmol/h)[13], and increases with sham feeding. Its effectiveness is thought to be increased by acting in an unstirred layer. Luminal acid stimulates gastric alkali secretion up to ten-fold, a response mediated by endogenous production of prostaglandins, humoral factors, and possibly, by nervous mechanisms[14]. However, the pH gradient would be overwhelmed at a luminal pH of greater than 1.5, and other methods of resisting hydrogen ion probably exist. It has recently been suggested that there is a movement of hydrogen ion against its gradient through the mucus due to a standing gradient of sodium ion across the mucus[15].

The Mucosal Barrier and Repair

Particularly in the fundic region, the gastric mucosa is covered by a tight epithelium whose function is thought to be the containment of hydrogen ion within the lumen. In rats and dogs, removal of surface mucus causes a 50% increase in the rate of hydrogen ion permeation. Because of its greater phospholipid content and hence hydrophobic properties[16], removal of the intracellular mucus caused a 2.5-fold rise in permeation, but mucosal resistance on its own was still much greater than that of a saline control[17]. When the mucus barrier is disrupted, as it can be by such agents as aspirin, ethanol and bile salts, the expected change in mucosal permeation enables hydrogen ion to diffuse in large amounts into the mucosa and sodium and potassium to move into the lumen – the back-diffusion phenomena. Experimentally, these changes result in damage to the gastric mucosa and the formation of erosions and ulceration. However, the gastric epithelium is capable of rapid reconstitution after acute damage[18]. Thirty minutes after rendering the surface epithelium necrotic, the epithelial surface had been reconstituted by a process of spreading of the cells which appeared at the necks of residual glands.

Mucosal Blood Flow

Just as an acute reduction in blood supply has been implicated in the aetiology of stress ulcers, so also has the suggestion been made that a chronic reduction in blood supply may predispose towards chronic ulceration. There is no clear evidence for this in duodenal ulcers, but arterial injection studies *in vitro* have demonstrated that the lesser curve of the stomach is a watershed of relatively poor vascularity compared with the highly vascular anterior and posterior walls of the stomach on each side of the lesser curve. This factor could indeed be part of the reason for the usual location of a gastric ulcer.

Whatever causes the breakdown of the tissue, the real question is, what prevents an ulcer in the gastroduodenal epithelium from healing? After all, that particular epithelium regenerates particularly rapidly; so much so that in man the lining cells are completely replaced every four or five days.

Virchow[19] proposed that mucosal blood flow had a role in maintaining the integrity of the mucosal barrier. The exposure of the gastric mucosa to various ulcerogens is accompanied by a compensatory increase in mucosal blood flow, and a reduction of the mucosal microcirculation results in an enhancement of lesion formation[20]. In rats with ligated stomachs and interrupted blood circulation, filling the stomach with absolute ethanol destroyed the mucosa within minutes. With intact circulation, the mucosa remained macroscopically normal or developed lesions, and after 30 minutes, 84% of the mucosa was reconstituted in the presence of the alcohol[21]. Two mechanisms by which mucosal blood flow aids this process have been proposed: the maintenance of adequate tissue oxygenation for repair and renewal, and the removal or buffering of 'escaped' luminal acid, resulting in an alkaline 'tide' on active gastric secretion. Kivilaakso[22] measured gastric pH and gastric mucosal blood flow in dogs, which were in shock, and found a fall in the pH that coincided with the development of lesions. The addition of HCO_3 prevented the lesion formation. They concluded that impaired capacity of the mucosa to dispose of hydrogen ion, rather than tissue anoxia, placed the mucosa in jeopardy. They also found that an actively secreting mucosa was able to resist mucosal damage much better than a resting one. Vascular changes and mucosal ischaemia may therefore be important in the pathogenesis of stress and drug-induced peptic ulcer, but its role in chronic ulceration is unknown.

Humoral Factors

In a review article on gastric cytoprotection, Konturek[23] cited the role of prostaglandins in maintaining the protective capacity of the mucosa. Prostaglandins are derivatives of 20-carbon-chain unsaturated fatty acids, and a major stimulus to their synthesis is any perturbation of cell membranes, such as the attempt to disrupt the mucosa or to collect its products. Most cells do not store prostaglandins, but produce it on demand. There are, therefore considerable problems in the interpretation of data about prostaglandins, but the consensus of opinion is that they are in some way cyto-protective i.e. they can cause a general enhancement of the mucosal resistance to damage[24]. For instance, most animal studies show that E prostaglandins prevent or reduce alterations in hydrogen ion permeability to aspirin, bile or alcohol. Prostaglandins have been shown to stimulate bicarbonate secretion, mucus glycoproteins, mucosal growth and increased mucosal blood flow, and they alter mucus structure. Irritants will stimulate prostaglandin synthesis, and endogenous synthesis may inhibit acid secretion. Also, long-term prostaglandin treatment leads to gastric mucosal hyperplasia in humans, and it is therefore conceivable that protection and repair are one and the same process.

However, it is unclear whether sufferers of peptic ulcer have any lack of protective factors. For instance, in one study, duodenal ulcer patients had no postcibal rise in prostaglandin content in contrast to controls, but the antecibal prostaglandin levels were higher in the DU. Prostaglandins appear to be a prime factor in mucosal protection, but an overriding role for them has not yet appeared, and peptic ulcer sufferers have not yet been shown to be particularly lacking in prostaglandins.

Pathophysiology of Mucosal Defences

Acute insult to the gastric mucosal barrier by such drugs as aspirin and alcohol can lead to the disruption of the barrier and hence susceptibility to attack by acid, pepsin or bile. Non-steroidal anti-inflammatory drugs can inhibit alkali and mucus secretion, and they appear to be involved in the aetiology of chronic gastric ulceration when they have been taken over a long period of time[25]. These drugs inhibit alkali and mucus secretion, as well as endogenous prostaglandin synthesis, and so a case can be made for their action being an aetiological factor in gastric ulcer.

Bile refluxing from the duodenum into the stomach is commonly reported to be in greater concentrations in the stomachs of gastric ulcer patients than in controls. Bile salts in quite low concentrations have been found to inhibit alkali secretion in mammalian fundic mucosa in vitro[26], and studies in man have shown that sodium taurocholate, a bile salt, inhibits alkali secretion and prostaglandin release[27]. High concentrations of bile acids cause mucosal damage. Since bile acid concentrations are reported to be higher in gastric ulcer patients than in controls or duodenal ulcer patients[28,29], it is tempting to attribute some gastric ulcers to refluxing bile. This contention is supported by the finding of lower acid secretion rates in gastric ulcer patients, supposedly due to a reduction in parietal cells because of mucosal damage. However, these patients tend to be old and female, and since maximal gastric secretion at least is influenced by age and height, it may be that the amount of bile is essentially normal, but is diluted in a less than normal volume. The question then is whether their gastric secretion is impaired at all? The maximal gastric secretion of gastric ulcer patients is found to be less the further from the pylorus. Indeed, pre-pyloric ulcers tend to have higher than normal maximal gastric secretion, in the very area where mucosal damage would be expected to be greatest.

Peptic ulcer patients have a greater amount of pepsin1, and it has recently been shown[30] that this fraction of pepsin has an increased mucolytic activity with respect to pepsin 3, and in particular will degrade gastric mucus at the higher pH values of 4 and above. There have also been reports of defects in the mucus of peptic ulcer patients, particularly those with gastric ulcer. These findings may be additional important factors.

In rats with cysteamine-induced duodenal ulcer, neutralization has been found to be reduced, in conjunction with deficiencies in two enzymes; a bicarbonate-sensitive ATPase and carbonic anhydrase[31]. Ahlquist[32] has shown that the production of prostaglandins in duodenal mucosal biopsies after acid stimulation is lower in ulcer patients than in normal subjects and Hillier et al[33] have found 50% reductions in certain prostaglandins in DU. The alkali secretion of the duodenum is mediated by endogenous prostaglandins and hence any defect here, coupled with an increased acid load, would be of particular importance. Konturek[34] though, found no deficiency in the generation of gastric or duodenal prostaglandins in duodenal ulcer patients.

In seven healthy smokers, the release of prostaglandin E_2 by the gastric mucosa after smoking three cigarettes was found to be significantly reduced[35]. Although the gastric bicarbonate output of duodenal ulcer patients under conditions of submaximal acid secretion has been found to be similar to that of controls[36], pancreatic bicarbonate secretion by duodenal ulcer patients in response to duodenal acidification is higher than normal[37]. In animal studies, intravenously-infused nicotine has been found to depress secretin-stimulated pancreatic and biliary secretion of fluid and bicarbonate, the degree of inhibition being related to the dose of nicotine. In man, secretin-stimulated pancreatic volume and bicarbonate output is acutely depressed in light smokers compared to non-smokers, and chronically depressed in heavy smokers, though this finding has not been confirmed. McCloy[38], for example, found no change in duodenal pH after smoking cigarettes. Neither did they find any difference in duodenal pH between controls and duodenal ulcer patients after a test meal. Shulze[39] found a significant association between duodenal ulcer and reduced exocrine pancreatic function in patients presenting with dyspeptic symptoms, and who were primarily suspected of having chronic pancreatitis.

EPIDEMIOLOGICAL AND GENETIC CONSIDERATIONS

The evidence that duodenal ulcer is a heterogenous condition has been steadily accumulating[40]. That is, the end result, an ulcer, may arise from several different factors acting together or singly. One factor thought to differentiate some duodenal ulcer patients from others is hypersensitivity to gastrin, and others are early and late onset, familial history and abnormally large maximal gastric secretion. Lam and Koo[41] sought to examine the relationship of these factors in 200 endoscopically proven duodenal ulcer patients and 38 controls. Early and late onset were classified by the division of age 30 years, and previous studies had indicated that early onset DU were more familial and had a normal population level of blood group O. Gastric hypersecretion was defined as being greater than 2 standard deviations above the normal mean, after weight correction. For each subject the dose of pentagastrin required for half maximal acid output was calculated from the response to different doses of pentagastrin. Compared to the controls, the results signified a greater sensitivity to pentagastrin in the DU. Among patients with normal acid output, pentagastrin sensitivity was greater in late onset and positive family history sub-groups. For those patients with abnormally high acid output, the reverse was true, with greater sensitivity to gastrin being found in those with early onset and negative family history. Environmental and genetic factors were thought to be at work in both groups. Another paper that recently examined hypersecretion of gastric acid in Finnish families[42] found that 4% of the sample (from the population at large) had gastric hypersecretion. They differed from the whole sample with regard to a high prevalence of signs of duodenal ulcer disease, of high serum pepsinogen, of blood group O and lack of gastric antibodies, and of high serum gastrin levels. The absence of hypersecretors in the children of the parent hypersecretors seemed to rule out the possibility of a dominant Mendelian inheritance.

Another study of gastrin responses in duodenal ulcer patients[43] sought to examine the concept that the subgroup of DU with hypergastrinaemia and acid hypersecretion had a defective acid inhibition of gastrin release. They compared gastrin and acid secretion responses to intragastric instillation of a mixture of amino acids in normal and G-cell hyperfunction patients. The results did not support the idea of impaired acid inhibition, but rather pointed to increased sensitivity of the G-cell to amino acid stimulation. This effect, combined with enhanced gastrin response to feeding and an increased sensitivity to circulating gastrins in the DU may have a long-lasting trophic influence on the parietal cell mass, and hence lead to increased acid secretory capacity.

Epidemiologically, there have been some very interesting new developments in peptic ulcer disease. In Hong Kong, for instance, there has been an increasing incidence over the past decade. Langman[44] has reviewed the trends in the United Kingdom, and using the most useful guide to prevalence, that of perforated ulcer rates, has found a steady fall over the period 1958 to 1977. There was a relatively greater fall in overall admission rates compared to admissions for perforation, and if it is assumed that the ratio of perforation to non-perforation remains constant, this would suggest a change in management. However, the fall antedates the introduction of

H_2 antagonists by some 10 years. Taken overall, the rates of admission for perforated peptic ulcer in England and Wales have fallen dramatically, particularly in the young and in men. However, there have been increases in perforated gastric ulcer in women over 75, and in perforated duodenal ulcer in women over 65. Langman concluded that these changes could not simply be ascribed to environmental influences, but it was more likely that younger individuals are less likely to be exposed to, or more likely to be resistant to, predisposing factors. Why these factors should demonstrate a sex bias remains unclear. Duodenal ulcer is mainly a disease of males, though the sex ratio worldwide is variable, being even more male-dominated in Third World countries. In the United States[45], data for the years 1957–81 demonstrate a decrease in the male: female ratios for perceived peptic ulcer and hospitalization rates. Hospitalization rates had decreased for both sexes, whilst perceived ulcer had decreased for men, but increased for women, and there was also an increased hospitalization rate for gastric ulcer in women over 65. The authors concluded that cigarette smoking has a time pattern similar to that of peptic ulcer hospitalization and mortality, and was worth further investigation. A similar time pattern has been observed for the consumption of linoleic acid[46], as vegetable oil, and the ability of such polyunsaturated fatty acids to stimulate greatly the production of prostaglandins in the stomach, when administered intragastrically, has suggested the hypothesis that they have contributed to the decrease in peptic ulcer.

This decline in incidence cannot be attributed to the introduction of H_2-blockers in 1977 since in both the United States and the UK, the decline preceded their introduction. The fall had been interpreted by Susser and Stein as a birth-cohort phenomena. Cohort effects are environmental effects which determine the fate of a generation (a birth-cohort) with respect to, in this case, peptic ulcer antecedent to the time when the ulcer occurred. Sonnenberg[47], in his analysis of cohort effect, considered the cohort phenomena to start at age 5 or below for both gastric and duodenal ulcers. He therefore ruled out such environmental factors as smoking or drug consumption. Opposed to this analysis are the observations on migrant workers from Southern Europe in Belgium, West Germany and Switzerland. In male migrant workers younger than 60, duodenal ulcer occurred twice as frequently as in the native population of the same age. Migrant workers older than 60(!) were not affected. The incidence of gastric ulcer in men and both ulcer types in women were the same as in the native population. A similar phenomenon has been reported from South Africa, where duodenal ulcer used to be rare in rural black communities, but is now becoming increasingly common in young urbanized males, mirroring the early finding in the UK of an increased incidence of DU in towns compared to the country.

A prospective study of the association between smoking, alcohol, coffee and familial factors and radiologically-diagnosed peptic ulcer has recently been carried out in North Norway, using 4081 dyspeptic patients[48]. They found, as others have before them, a statistically increased prevalence of peptic ulcer disease in relatives of patients with peptic ulcer, with a stronger association for gastric ulcer in women (relative risk 2.07). No association was found with coffee, consumption being significantly lower in peptic ulcer patients, and smoking was more frequently seen in patients with duodenal ulcer than in patients with gastric ulcer. Furthermore, significantly more smokers were noted among patients with duodenal ulcers than among their controls. The relative risk from smoking was increased in both ulcer groups and in both sexes. In addition, in men, there was a statistically significant positive correlation between the amount of tobacco used and the relative risk, increasing up to a value of 2.63 for smokers on 20 or more cigarettes per day. No association was found with alcohol. Indeed, in patients with duodenal ulcer, the number of alcohol users was significantly lower than in the control group, perhaps as a response to their ulcer.

Stress is commonly thought to be associated with peptic ulcer. Urbanization and army training have been found to have increased incidences of duodenal ulcer, and so support the hypothesis of the role of stress. However, air traffic controllers do not suffer an increased incidence of duodenal ulcer and stressful life events do not appear to be risk factors for the exacerbation of symptoms in duodenal ulcer patients[49], nor do they perceive that their reaction to life events are more severe than non-sufferers[50].

Birth-cohort phenomena and increased incidence amongst relatives are suggestive of a genetic component to peptic ulcer. Blood group O predominates in patients with duodenal ulcer, and blood group O and non-secretor status are associated with an increased risk of DU. There are also well-defined genetic syndromes that feature duodenal ulcer disease. Multiple endocrine adenomatosis is an autosomal dominant disorder characterized by pituitary, parathyroid, and pancreatic adenomas, the latter secreting excess gastrin leading to gross acid hypersecretion and eventually the Zollinger–Ellison syndrome. Excessive histamine, as found in systemic mastocytosis, can also lead to gastric hypertrophy, acid hypersecretion and duodenal ulcer. Hyperpepsinogenaemia, associated with a pachydermoperiostosis syndrome, can also produce duodenal ulcer. Hyperpepsinogenaemia I has also been found to be a sub-clinical marker for duodenal ulcer in two large families. Healthy first-degree relatives of hyperpepsinogenaemic duodenal ulcer patients have serum pepsinogen values intermediate between the patients and the segregation of the hyperpepsinogenaemia is consistent with autosomal dominant inheritance in many families[51]. Such a result has also been found in an Indian sample[52].

In summary, peptic ulcer, and duodenal ulcer in particular, seem to present with a wealth of pathophysiological and genetic defects, hence giving rise to the multi-factorial hypothesis. However, pathophysiological disturbances are not necessarily of aetiological significance and may only be a consequence of the disease, not a precursor. Wormsley[53], pursuing this argument, pointed to the more direct evidence of the ulcerogenic effect of aspirin, nitrile derivatives and the very high titres of antibodies to herpes simplex virus, type 1, found in some patients with duodenal ulcer. More recently[54,55], *Campylobacter pyloridis*, a spiral bacterium on gastric mucosa, has been found to be associated with gastritis and duodenal ulcer.

It may therefore be that the solution to the aetiology of peptic ulcer lies in the quest for a variety of exogenous, environmental influences, perhaps acting on a genetically primed individual. The exogenous factors could, of course, increase the attacking factors, decrease the protective factors, or both.

REFERENCES

1. Marrane, G. C. and Silen, W. (1984). Pathogenesis, diagnosis and treatment of acute gastric mucosal lesions. *Clin. Gastroenterol.*, **13**, 635–650
2. Oi, M., Oshida, K. and Sugimura, S. (1959). The location of gastric ulcer. *Gastroenterology*, **36**, 45–56
3. Ruding, R. (1967) Gastric ulcer and antral border. *Surgery*, **61**, 495–497
4. Kay, A. W. (1953). Effect of large doses of histamine on gastric secretion of HCl. *Br. Med. J.*, **2**, 77–80
5. Baron, J. H. (1969). Lean body mass, gastric acid and peptic ulcer. *Gut*, **10**, 637–642
6. Whitfield, P. F. and Hobsley, M. (1979). A standardized technique for the performance of accurate gastric secretion studies. *Agents Actions*, **9**, 327–332
7. Hassan, M. A. and Hobsley, M. (1971). The accurate assessment of maximal gastric secretion in control subjects and patients with duodenal ulcer. *Br. J. Surg.*, **58**, 171–179
8. Lam, S. K., Hasan, M., Sircus, W., Wong, J., Ong, G. B. and Prescott, R. J. (1980). Comparison of maximal acid output and gastrin response to meals in Chinese and Scottish normal and duodenal ulcer subjects. *Gut*, **21**, 324–328
9. Parente, F., Lazzaroni, M., Ornela, S., Stefani, B. and Bianchi Porro, G. (1985). Cigarette smoking, gastric acid secretion and serum pepsinogen 1 concentration in DU patients. *Gut*, **26**, 1327–1332
10. Whitfield, P. F. and Hobsley, M. (1985). Maximal gastric secretion in smokers and non-smokers with duodenal ulcer. *Br. J. Surg.*, **72**, 955–957
11. McQueen, S., Allen, A. and Garner, A. (1984). Measurement of gastric and duodenal mucus gel thickness. In Allen, A., Flemstrom, G., Garner, A., Silen, W. and Turnberg, L. A. (eds.) *Mechanisms of mucosa protection in the upper gastrointestinal tract.* pp. 215–219. (New York: Raven Press)
12. Flemstrom, G. and Garner, A. (1982). Gastroduodenal HCO_3 trans-

port: characteristics and proposed role in acidity regulation and mucosal protection by the normal human stomach *in vivo*. *Am. J. Physiol.*, **242**, G183–G193

13. Rees, W. D. W., Botham, D. and Turnberg, L. A. (1982). A demonstration of bicarbonate production by the normal human stomach *in vivo*. *Dig. Dis. Sci.*, **27**, 961–966
14. Heylings, J. R., Garner, A. and Flemstrom, G. (1984). Regulation of gastroduodenal HCO_3 transport by luminal acid in the frog *in vitro*. *Am. J. Physiol.*, **246**, G235–G242
15. Smith, G. W., Tasman-Jones, C., Wiggins, P. M. and Len, S. P. (1985). Pig gastric mucosa: A one-way barrier for hydrogen. *Gastroenterology*, **89**, 1313–1318
16. Hills, B. A., Butler, B. D. and Lichtenberger, L. M. (1983). Gastric mucosal barrier: hydrophobic lining to the lumen of the stomach. *Am. J. Physiol.*, **244**, G561–G568
17. Slomianey, B. L., Piasech, A., Sarosek, J. and Solemney, A. (1985). The role of surface and intracellular mucus in gastric mucosal protection against hydrogen ion. *Scand. J. Gastroenterol.*, **20**, 1191–1196
18. Rutten, M. J. and Ito, S. (1983). Morphology and electrophysiology of guinea-pig gastric mucosal repair *in vitro*. *Am J. Physiol.*, **244**, G171–G183
19. Virchow, R. (1853). Historisches, Kritisches und Positives zur lehre der Unterleibsaffektion. *Virchows Arch. A. Path. Anat. Histol.*, **5**, 632–650
20. Ritchie, W. P. (1975). Acute gastric mucosal damage induced by bile salts, acid and ischaemia. *Gastroenterology*, **18**, 699–707
21. Ito, S. and Lacy, E. R. (1986). Morphology of rat gastric mucosal damage, defense, and restitution in the presence of luminal ethanol. *Gastroenterology*, **88**, 250–260
22. Kivilaasko, E. (1981). High plasma HCO_3 protects gastric mucosa against acute ulceration in the rat. *Gastroenterology*, **81**, 921–927
23. Konturek, S. J. (1985). Gastric cytoprotection. *Scand. J. Gastroenterol.*, **20**, 543–553
24. Johannsen, C., Ay, A., Befrits, R., Smedfors, B. and Uribe, A. (1985). Protection of the gastro-duodenal mucosa by prostaglandins. *Scand. J. Gastroenterol. Suppl.*, **110**, 41–43
25. Piper, D. W., McIntosh, J. H., Ariotti, D. E., Fenton, B. H. and MacLennan, R. (1981). Analgesic ingestion and chronic peptic ulcer. *Gastroenterology*, **80**, 427–432
26. Rees, W. D. W., Garner, A., Turnberg, L. and Gillroy, L. C. (1982). Studies of acid and alkaline secretion by rabbit gastric fundus *in vitro*: effect of low concentrations of sodium taurocholate. *Gastroenterology*, **83**, 435–440
27. Rees, W. D. W., Warhurst, G. and Turnberg, L. A. (1982). Studies of bicarbonate secretion by the normal human stomach *in vitro*: effect of sodium taurocholate and aspirin. *Gastroenterology*, **82**, 1158 (abstract)
28. Gotthard, R., Bodemar, G., Tjadermo, M., Tobiasson, P. and Walan, A. (1985). High gastric bile acid concentrations in pre-pyloric ulcer patients. *Scand. J. Gastroenterol.*, **20**, 437–446

29. Rydning, A. and Berstad, A. (1985). Intragastric bile acid concentration in healthy subjects and in patients with gastric and duodenal ulcer and the influence of fiber-enriched wheat bran in patients with gastric ulcer. *Scand. J. Gastroenterol.*, **20**, 801–804

30. Pearson, J. P., Ward, R., Allen, A. A., Roberts, N. B. and Taylor, W. H. (1986). Mucus degradation by pepsin: comparison of mucolytic activity of human pepsin 1 and pepsin 3: implications in peptic ulceration. *Gut*, **27**, 243–248

31. Stiel, D., Murray, D. J. and Peters, T. J. (1983). Mucosal enzyme activities with special reference to enzymes implicated in bicarbonate secretion in the duodenum of rats with cysteamine-induced ulcers. *Clin. Sci.*, **64**, 341–347

32. Ahlquist, D. A., Pozois, R. R., Zinsmuster, A. R. and Malagdelada, J. R. (1982). Duodenal prostaglandin synthesis and acid load in health and in duodenal ulcer disease. *Gastroenterology*, **85**, 522–528

33. Hillier, K., Smith, C. C., Jewell, R., Arther, M. J. P. and Ross, G. (1985). Duodenal mucosa synthesis of prostaglandins in duodenal ulcer disease. *Gut*, **26**, 237–240

34. Konturek, S. J., Obtulowicz, W., Sito, E., Olesky, J., Wildon, S. and Kiec-Dembinska, A. (1981). Distribution of prostaglandins in gastric and duodenal mucosa of healthy subjects and duodenal ulcer patients: effect of aspirin and paracetamol. *Gut*, **22**, 283–289

35. McCready, D. R., Clark, L. and Cohen, M. M. (1985). Cigarette smoking reduces human gastric luminal prostaglandin E2. *Gut*, **26**, 1192–1196

36. Feldman, M. and Barrett, C. C. (1985). Gastric bicarbonate secretion in patients with duodenal ulcer. *Gastroenterology*, **88**, 1205–1208

37. Isenberg, J. I., Cano, R. and Bloom, S. R. (1973). Effect of graded amounts of acid instilled into the duodenum on pancreatic bicarbonate secretion and plasma secretin in duodenal ulcer patients and normal subjects. *Gastroenterology*, **72**, 6–8

38. McCloy, R. F., Greenberg, G. R. and Baron, J. H. (1984). Duodenal pH in health and duodenal ulcer disease: effect of a meal, Coca-Cola, smoking and Cimetidine. *Gut*, **25**, 386–392

39. Schulze, S., Thosgaard, P. N., Jorensen, M. J., Mollman, K.-M. and Rune, S. J. (1983). Association between duodenal bulb ulceration and reduced exocrine pancreatic function. *Gut*, **24**, 78–83

40. Rotter, J. I. and Rimoin, D. L. (1979). Peptic ulcer disease – a heterogenous group of disorders? *Gastroenterology*, **73**, 604–607

41. Lam, S. K. and Koo, J. (1985). Gastrin sensitivity in duodenal ulcer. *Gut*, **26**, 485–490

42. Kekki, M., Sipponen, P. and Suirala, M. (1985). Hypersecretion of gastric acid in a representative Finnish family sample. *Scand. J. Gastroenterol.*, **20**, 478–484

43. Cooper, R. G., Dockray, G. J., Colam, J. and Walker, R. (1985). Acid and gastrin response during intragastric titration in normal subjects and duodenal ulcer patients with G-cell hyperfunction. *Gut*, **26**, 232–236

44. Langman, M. J. S. (1984). Recent changes in the pattern of chronic

digestive disease in the United Kingdom. *Postgrad. Med. J.*, **60**, 733–736

45. Kurata, J. H., Haile, B. M. and Elashoff, J. D. (1985). Sex differences in peptic ulcer disease. *Gastroenterology*, **80**, 96–100

46. Hollander, D. and Tarnawski, A. (1986). Dietary essential fatty acids and the decline in peptic ulcer disease – a hypothesis. *Gut*, **27**, 239–242

47. Sonnenberg, A. (1985). Geographic and temporal variation in the occurrence of peptic ulcer disease. *Scand. J. Gastroenterol., Suppl.* **110**, 11–24

48. Ostensen, H., Gudmundsen, T. E., Ostensen, M., Burhol, P. G. and Bonnevie, O. (1985). Smoking, alcohol, coffee and familial factors: Any association with peptic ulcer disease. *Scand. J. Gastroenterol.*, **20**, 1227–1235

49. Piper, D. W., McIntosh, J. H., Ariotti, D. E. et al. (1981). Life events and chronic duodenal ulcer: a case control study. *Gut*, **22**, 1011–1017

50. McIntosh, J. H., Nasing, R. W., McNeil, D., Coates, C., Mitchell, H. and Piper, D. W. (1985). Perception of life event stress in patients with chronic duodenal ulcer. A comparison of the rating of life events by duodenal ulcer patients and community controls. *Scand. J. Gastroenterol.*, **20**, 563–568

51. Rotter, J. I., Somes, J. Q., Samloff, I. M. et al. (1979). Duodenal ulcer disease associated with elevated serum pepsinogen I – an inherited autosomal dominant disorder. *N. Engl. J. Med.*, **300**, 63–65

52. Habibulbah, C. M., Mujahid Ali, M., Ishaq, M., Prasad, R., Pratap, B. and Saleem, Y. (1984). Study of duodenal ulcer disease in 100 families using total serum pepsinogen as a genetic marker. *Gut*, **25**, 1380–1383

53. Wormsley, K. G. (1983). Duodenal ulcer: does pathophysiology equal aetiology? *Gut*, **24**, 775–780

54. Price, A. B., Levi, J., Dolby, J. M., Dunscombe, P. L., Smith, A., Clark, J. and Stephenson, M. L. (1985). *Campylobacter pyloridis* in peptic ulcer disease: microbiology, pathology and scanning electron microscopy. *Gut*, **26**, 1183–1188

55. Rathbone, B. J., Wyatt, J. I., Wordsey, B. W., Shires, S. E., Trejdosiewicz, L. K., Heatley, R. V., Losowsky, M. S. (1986). Systemic and local antibody responses to gastric *Campylobacter pyloridis* in non-ulcer dyspepsia. *Gut*, **27**, 642–647

2

OESOPHAGITIS

A. J. M. WATSON and M. J. G. FARTHING

INTRODUCTION

Oesophagitis is one of the commonest gastrointestinal disorders and is encountered by both general practitioners and hospital specialists alike. Its principal symptom is retrosternal burning pain or 'heartburn' which results from the reflux of gastric acid into the oesophagus causing mucosal inflammation (reflux oesophagitis). In many patients reflux will not be severe enough to cause inflammatory changes in the mucosa but will be sufficient to cause symptoms and the term 'reflux disease' is often used to refer to this more general condition.

It is difficult to estimate the prevalence of reflux oesophagitis as many patients consider heartburn normal and do not seek medical attention, while in others, particularly the elderly, it is asymptomatic. A survey of hospital employees showed that 7% experienced daily heartburn and 36% had this symptom once a month[1]. Reflux oesophagitis can affect all age-groups including young children and the elderly, and is particularly common during pregnancy when as many as 25% of women have daily symptoms[1].

Some patients present with atypical symptoms mimicking

cardiac pain, while others, particularly children, present with pulmonary symptoms. Although the majority of patients obtain symptomatic relief from simple medical measures, in some, especially the elderly, oesophagitis may progress despite symptomatic relief and result in stricture formation or haemorrhage. In others (about 5–10%), medical measures fail to relieve the symptoms and surgery is required.

THE ANTI-REFLUX BARRIER

Before considering the pathogenesis of oesophagitis it is important to have a clear understanding of normal mechanisms preventing reflux of gastric contents into the oesophagus. At the lower end of the oesophagus there is an anti-reflux barrier formed by the lower oesophageal sphincter (LOS). There are two major contributory mechanisms which produce the LOS, one physiological and the other mechanical (Figures 2.1 and 2.2).

Physiological Sphincter

There is no visible band of muscle forming a sphincter as in the pylorus or anus, but manometric studies reveal a high pressure zone about 4 cm long, situated partly in the thorax and partly in the abdomen. This zone is distinct from the rest of the oesophagus because it generates active tone while at rest which results in a squeeze of 15 mmHg creating a physiological sphincter[2]. The intragastric pressure is zero most of the time except just after meals when it will rise for a few seconds to 10–15 mmHg resulting in the reflux of small quantities of gastric contents into the oesophagus. This occurs in healthy subjects without symptoms of oesophagitis and so must be considered a normal phenomenon. The physiological sphincter is under neurological control via the vagus which increases the pressure and humoral control by many gut peptides and other

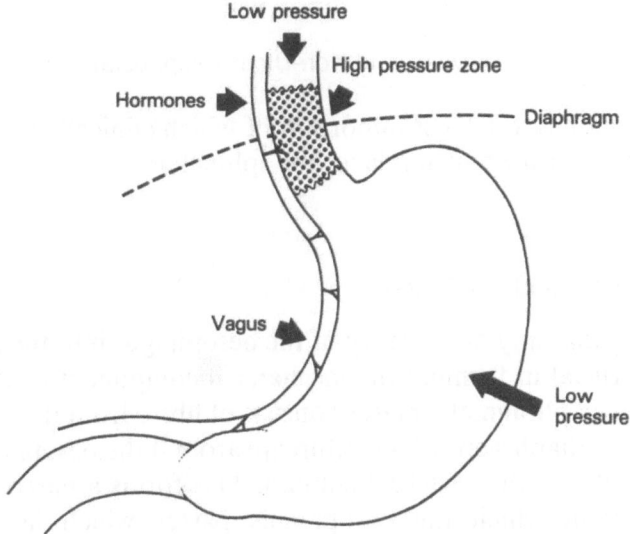

Figure 2.1   The anti-reflux barrier: the physiological sphincter

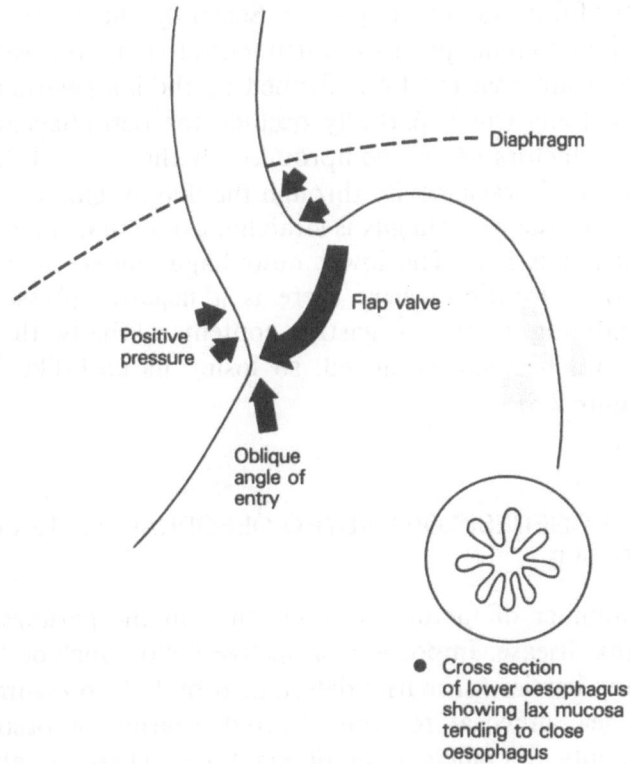

Figure 2.2   The anti-reflux barrier: the mechanical sphincter

hormones, the most important of which clinically is probably progesterone which relaxes the sphincter.

Mechanical Sphincter

The anatomy of the entry of the oesophagus into the stomach is crucial in forming the mechanical component of the LOS. The diaphragmatic hiatus consists of fibres from the right crus of the diaphragm which bifurcate around the oesophagus and insert into the vertebral column. This forms a narrow tunnel through which the oesophagus passes which incidentally widens with increasing age. A number of factors are of importance in forming the mechanical sphincter. First, is the oblique angle of entry of the oesophagus into the stomach which results in the formation of a flap valve. Secondly, there is the positive intra-abdominal pressure which tends to close this valve. Finally, a mucosal rosette is formed by the lax gastric mucosal form folds which partially occlude the oesophageal lumen. These factors are all compromised if the stomach herniates into the thoracic cavity through the diaphragm. The oblique entry of the oesophagus is straightened so that the flap valve function is lost. The lower oesophagus moves to an intra-thoracic location where there is a negative pressure, thus facilitating reflux of gastric contents. Finally the gastric mucosa becomes stretched, so losing its cork-like function (Figure 2.3).

PATHOGENESIS OF GASTRO-OESOPHAGEAL REFLUX DISEASE

A number of factors are concerned in the pathogenesis of reflux disease. Important protective factors include the anti-reflux barrier (primarily determined by LOS pressure), oeso-phageal mucosal resistance, rapid clearing of oesophageal contents and efficient gastric emptying. There are also some

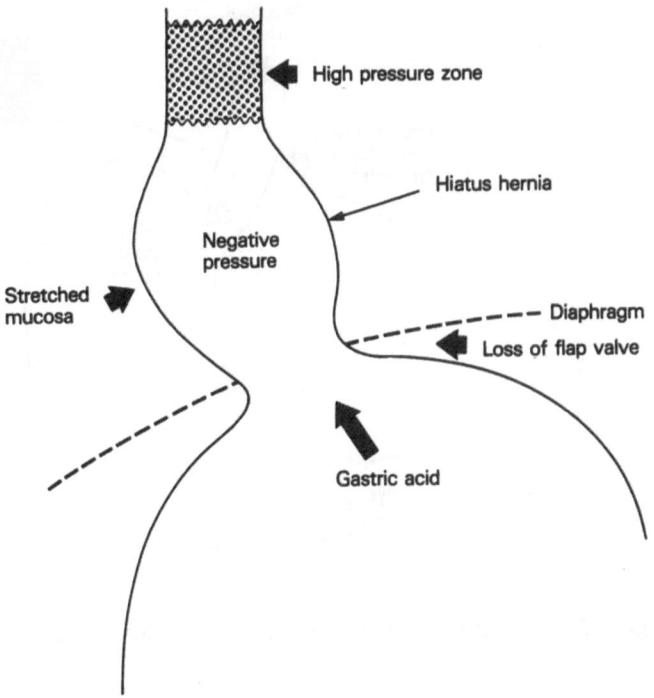

Figure 2.3   Disruption of the oesophageal sphincter by hiatus hernia

aggressive factors such as the pH of the gastric contents and reflux of alkaline duodenal fluid (Figure 2.4).

LOS Pressure

Until recently it was thought that the LOS pressure was not important in the pathogenesis of reflux disease because of the poor correlation between LOS pressure and clinical oesophageal reflux. However, the sphincter tone varies considerably during the day particularly after meals, alcohol, drugs including anticholinergics and cigarette smoking. This means that a single measurement of the LOS pressure may not be representative. This has been borne out by a recent study

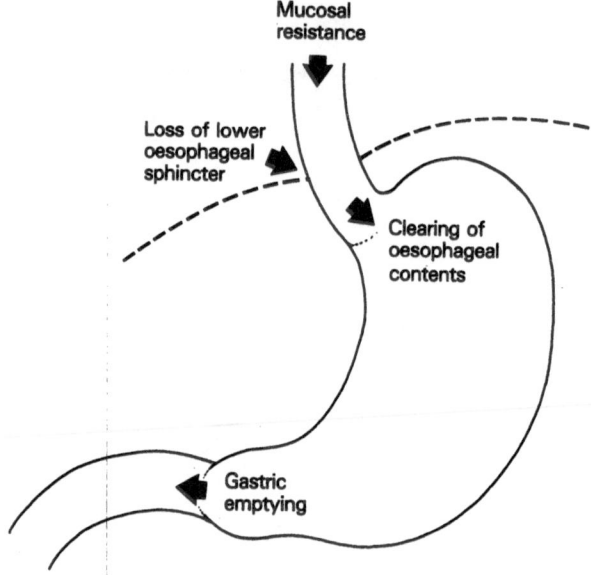

Figure 2.4 Factors in the pathogenesis of reflux disease

in which intra-oesophageal pH and pressure were monitored simultaneously over extended periods[4]. Reflux occurred primarily when the pressure was low; patients with low resting pressures had more episodes of reflux than controls. They also demonstrated transient relaxations of the sphincter with subsequent reflux in normal subjects. Thus, although the LOS pressure is variable, the mean pressure through the 24 hour period is crucial in preventing reflux and is one of the principal factors in preventing reflux disease.

A number of factors reduce the LOS pressure. Sphincter pressures progressively decrease during pregnancy under the influence of progesterone and are also decreased in women taking progesterone-containing oral contraceptives, and can even be reduced in the late stage of the menstrual cycle[5,6]. Smoking reduces LOS pressure by the anticholinergic action of nicotine[7]. Chocolate and coffee have also been shown to lower the pressure[8]. Systemic sclerosis will damage the muscle of the sphincter leading to severe reflux[9]. Vagotomy and surgery for achalasia can also directly damage the sphincter[10]. Hiatus hernia is found in many normal subjects and so cannot, in itself, be regarded as pathological[3]. Nevertheless, the presence of a hiatus hernia will lower the efficiency of the LOS and so is considered a factor in the pathogenesis of reflux disease.

Mucosal Resistance

The oesophageal mucosa is covered by squamous epithelium which is not, like the columnar gastric epithelium, resistant to hydrogen ions, pepsin or bile acids[11]. Exposure to these agents will change the potential difference across the mucosa and can also alter the enzyme content and structure of the mucosa[12]. The mechanisms which control the resistance of the mucosa to damage are not, as yet, fully understood but there is evidence that prostaglandins, particularly PGE_2, play an important role in the protection against injury.

Oesophageal Clearance

The oesophagus is cleared by peristalsis either after a swallow (primary peristalsis) or after distension (secondary peristalsis). Patients with reflux disease have defective peristalsis and require more swallows than normal individuals to raise an acid pH to neutral[13]. Oesophagitis can be particularly severe when peristalsis is defective as in systemic sclerosis. Recent work has shown that during sleep, acid clearance from the oesophagus is dependent on the number of swallows, which in turn is dependent on the patient arousing from sleep[14]. This study implies that if sleep arousal is depressed either by sedatives or alcohol, acid clearance will be impaired, thus increasing the likelihood of oesophagitis. This, however, has yet to be formally tested.

Gastric Acid and Gastric Emptying

Gastric factors have recently been realized to be of importance in the pathogenesis of reflux disease. The acidity of the gastric juice is of primary importance though the alkaline duodenal contents may also play a role, as oesophagitis can occur in achlorhydria or after total gastrectomy[15]. Some patients with reflux have delayed gastric emptying, thus increasing the potential for reflux. In addition, the anti-reflux barrier will be impaired while the stomach is distended with food[16].

SYMPTOMS OF GASTRO-OESOPHAGEAL REFLUX

The diagnosis of gastro-oesophageal reflux can be made in the majority of patients from the history, while there are no helpful physical signs.

Heartburn

This is the cardinal symptom of gastro-oesophageal reflux and is caused by the reflux of gastric contents over a sensitive oesophageal mucosa. It is a discomfort or pain, often burning in character, felt behind the sternum sometimes arising to the throat or radiating into the back. It occurs intermittently, being provoked by bending or stooping, lying flat, large meals or alcohol. It is quickly relieved by drinking water, milk or an antacid. Most people suffer from heartburn at some point in their lives but it is only when the symptom becomes frequent or disabling that it is considered pathological.

Other Varieties of Oesophageal Pain

Other types of pain may arise from the oesophagus probably due to motor abnormalities. They can be severe and are often described as 'gripping' or 'knife-like.' They may radiate into the neck, back or down both arms and can easily be mistaken for cardiac pain. A recent survey has shown that one-third of patients admitted to hospital with suspected myocardial infarction were actually suffering from gastro-oesophageal reflux[17].

Regurgitation

In some patients the effortless reflux of gastric contents (regurgitation) is a predominant symptom. Often patients will notice a bitter or sour taste in the mouth as a result.

Odynophagia

This is a transitory retrosternal pain on swallowing and is very suggestive of reflux disease.

Dysphagia

This is a sensation of delay of swallowed food at the lower end of the oesophagus. Although this usually indicates the presence of a stricture, it can be due to oesophagitis alone.

Haemorrhage

Bleeding from reflux oesophagitis accounts for about 4% of patients with gastrointestinal haemorrhage and can occur with either reflux oesophagitis alone or when oesophagitis is complicated by a peptic ulcer.

Respiratory Symptoms

There are patients whose chronic bronchitis or asthma appears to be exacerbated by reflux oesophagitis. Radio contrast material swallowed at night can be demonstrated in the lung the following day[15]. It is not yet clear how often reflux causes respiratory symptoms however, some patients can be found whose respiratory symptoms are helped by treatment for reflux.

Symptoms of Gastro-oesophageal Reflux in Infancy

Reflux in infancy is common but disappears as the child grows, presumably due to the narrowing of the diaphragmatic hiatus. The cardinal symptom at this age is frequent vomiting which can result in recurrent chest infections due to aspiration and undernutrition. Usually only conservative measures are required such as thickening the feeds and elevating the head when asleep.

COMPLICATIONS

Oesophagitis may have a number of complications including ulceration, columnar metaplasia (Barrett's syndrome), neoplasia and stricture formation.

Ulceration

This usually occurs at the junction of the oesophageal squamous mucosa and the gastric columnar mucosa (Figure 2.5). The symptoms are the same as those of reflux oesophagitis though they may be more severe and persistent. Ulcers may bleed and very occasionally perforate.

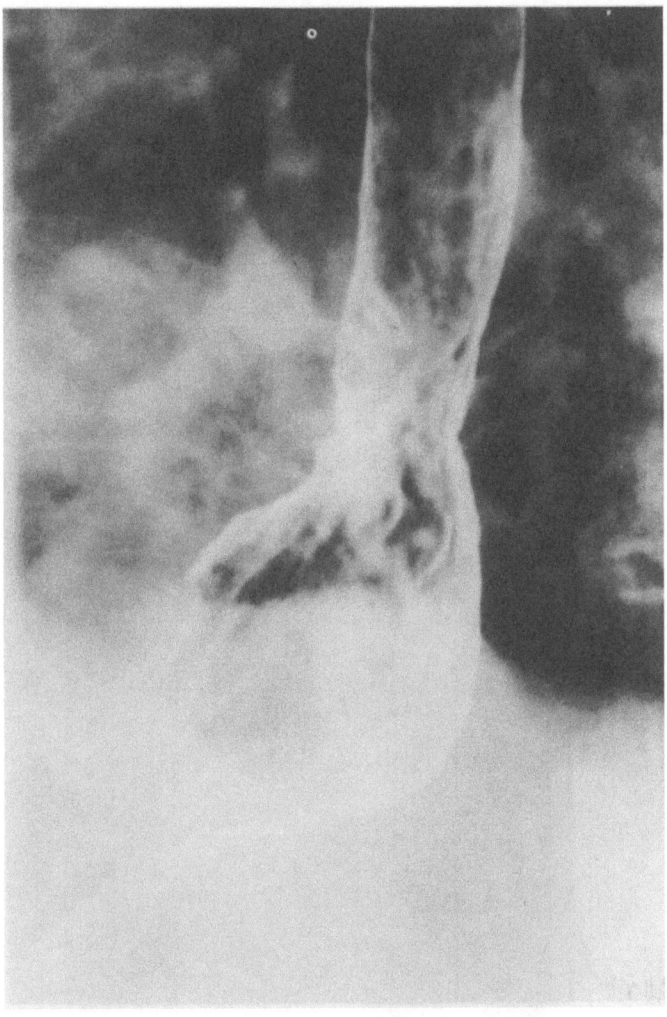

Figure 2.5   Radiograph from barium swallow examination showing ulceration in distal oesophagus

Columnar Metaplasia

In some patients with severe oesophagitis the squamous epithelium in the lower oesophagus may undergo metaplastic change to columnar epithelium (Barrett's syndrome)[18]. The demarcation between squamous and columnar epithelium, which can clearly be seen at endoscopy (the Z-line), occurs higher in the oesophagus than usual and extends proximally

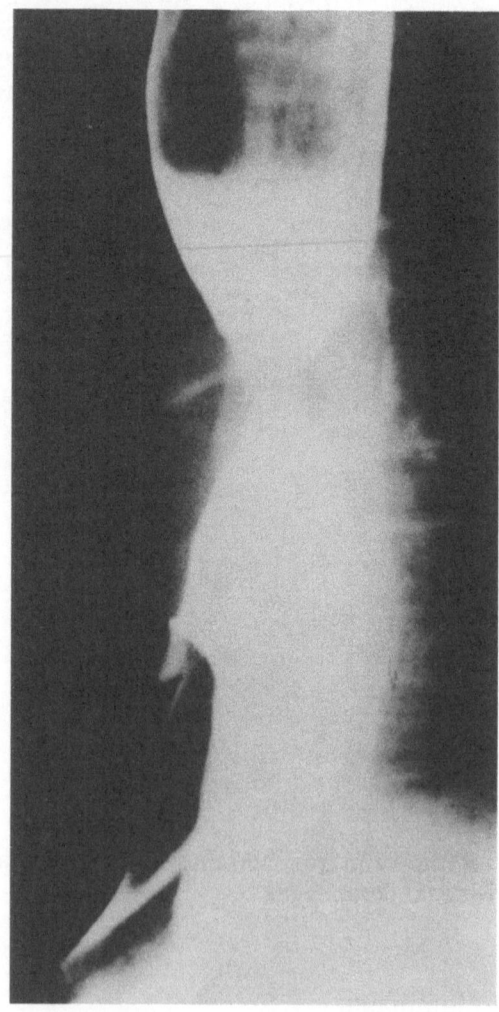

Figure 2.6   Radiograph showing Barrett's oesophagus with ulceration at the squamo-columnar mucosal junction

with time. This margin can become chronically ulcerated or can undergo stricture formation (Figure 2.6). The symptoms are no different from reflux disease but there is an increased incidence of carcinoma than in the normal oesophagus and thus Barrett's syndrome should be considered a pre-malignant condition. Barrett's syndrome occurs in about 8% of patients with reflux disease who have symptoms severe enough to be undergoing hospital investigation. The incidence of adeno-carcinoma is about 15% in this group of patients[19].

Stricture

Oesophageal reflux can cause stricture formation (Figure 2.7) but it is not clear how often this occurs. Severe prolonged oesophagitis will lead to strictures but about 50% of patients with strictures will deny any previous symptoms of reflux[15]. Conversely strictures can occur within a few weeks, especially after a prolonged placement of a large-bore nasogastric tube[15].

Dysphagia is the cardinal symptom of a stricture. The onset is usually gradual over many months or years. Dysphagia is generally for solids alone, only affecting liquids when the stricture is very tight or is obstructed by solid material. There may be pain when drinking hot liquids or alcohol due to associated mucosal inflammation around the stricture. If the onset of dysphagia is rapid or there is complete dysphagia for liquids as well as solids a malignant stricture should be suspected.

INVESTIGATIONS

There are now a bewildering array of tests available for the study of different aspects of gastro-oesophageal reflux. The *potential for reflux* can be assessed either by barium meal or

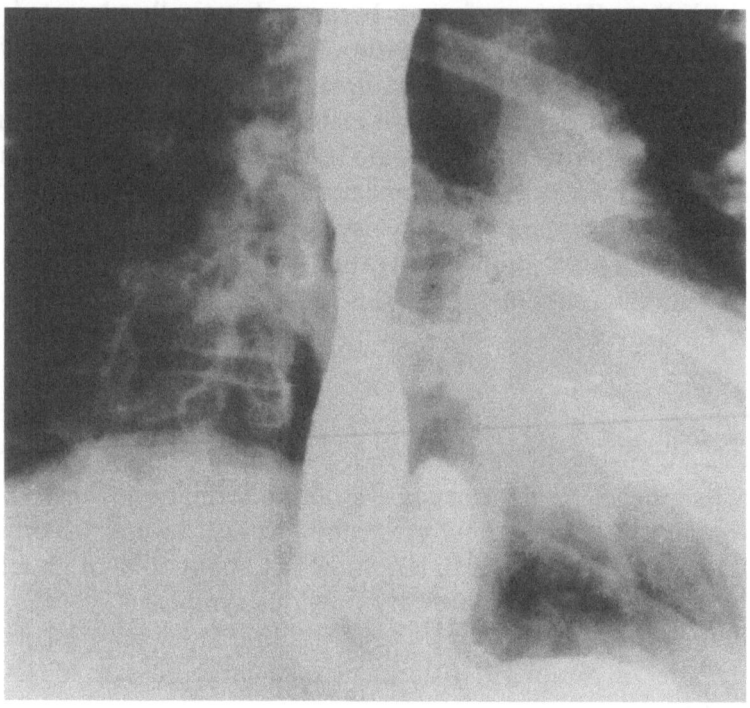

Figure 2.7   Radiograph showing a hiatus hernia, reflux oesophagitis and a benign stricture

measurement of the LOS pressure. *Damage to the oesophageal mucosa* may be judged by a barium meal, endoscopy and biopsy, or the Bernstein test. The *presence of actual reflux* can be detected again by barium meal, the standard acid reflux test, prolonged intraluminal pH monitoring or a scintiscan. Fortunately, in the majority of patients the symptoms are sufficiently clear-cut and the response to treatment rapid enough to render investigation superfluous; these patients can be properly managed without any investigation whatsoever. However, in patients in which the history is not diagnostic or the response to treatment is not adequate, investigation will be required.

Barium Swallow and Meal

This is the standard initial investigation for gastro-oeso-phageal reflux. Many patients with reflux disease have a hiatus hernia and it is sometimes assumed that there is a cause and effect relationship. One classic study into the relation between the symptoms of gastro-oesophageal reflux and hiatus hernia found that the incidence of hiatus hernia in asymptomatic controls was the same as in patients with chronic reflux symptoms[21]. Furthermore, the barium swallow and meal is a poor test for reflux and depends on the technique used by the radiologist. In a recent review it was shown to have an average sensitivity (diseased patient with positive test/diseased patient × 100%) as low as 40% but a specificity (non-diseased patients with a negative test/non-diseased patient × 100%) of 85%[22].

More recently the use of double-contrast radiographic techniques has allowed the mucosa to be examined in greater detail and this has been shown to have a sensitivity and specificity approaching 100% for moderate or severe oesophagitis, but is still insensitive to mild degrees of inflammation (22%)[23]. The radiographic signs of oesophagitis are marginal irregularity in the fully distended oesophagus, ulcerations, incomplete oeso-phageal distensibility and stricture formation.

The barium swallow and meal should be used in patients who have severe symptoms or whose symptoms are atypical, particularly to exclude other pathology which may be mim-icking reflux disease such as a gastric or duodenal ulcer. It is also useful to identify complications such as stricture for-mation or ulceration high in the oesophagus which may indi-cate Barrett's syndrome or a carcinoma at the cardia. Many patients will have a normal barium swallow and meal although this does not rule out reflux disease.

Upper Gastrointestinal Endoscopy

This is more expensive and possibly less comfortable than radiology but is nevertheless superior as it allows direct visual assessment of the mucosa and permits biopsies to be taken. In *moderate oesophagitis* there are round and longitudinal superficial ulcers or erosions, with a diffusely haemorrhagic mucosa, while in *severe oesophagitis* there are also deep punched-out ulcers and possibly oesophageal strictures[22]. The endoscopic criteria for *mild oesophagitis* are not well-defined. These include erythema, oedema of the mucosa with loss of visible blood vessels, mild friability and an increase in the irregularity of the junction between the oesophageal and gastric mucosa. These changes can be subjective and there is great inter-observer variation.

Oesophageal Histology

Some patients with definite reflux symptoms will have a macroscopically normal oesophageal mucosa on endoscopy but can be shown to have abnormalities on histological examination. In biopsies from normal subjects the dermal papillae extend less than halfway to the free luminal margin and the basal layer occupies less than 15% of the total thickness of the epithelium. In the lamina propria, polymorphonuclear leukocytes are never seen and eosinophils are uncommon[24]. In biopsies from patients with oesophagitis, the dermal papillae extend more than 50% to the surface and the basal layer occupies more than 15% of the epithelial thickness. Polymorphonuclear cells and eosinophils can be seen in the lamina propria in the more severe cases. These changes are most often seen in the lower 5 cm of the oesophagus[25].

Histological change should be highly discriminating in indicating whether reflux is damaging the mucosa or not, however in practice this is sometimes not so. The lesions are often patchy and can be missed. Also the small endoscopic biopsy forceps often do not take biopsies large enough for accurate interpretation by the histologist. One study showed that over 50% of these 'pinch' biopsies were uninterpretable when oesophagitis was mild or absent[26].

As biopsies are expensive to obtain, moderately uncomfortable and associated with a small risk they should be reserved for patients who are failing to respond to intensive medical therapy to assess whether there is objective evidence of failure and when Barrett's syndrome, stricture formation or carcinoma is suspected. As biopsies are often unreliable when changes are mild there seems little justification for their routine use.

Acid Perfusion (Bernstein) Test

The purpose of the acid perfusion test is to demonstrate the sensitivity of the lower oesophagus to acid. It is designed to provoke a symptom known to be oesophageal in origin so that this can be compared with the patients spontaneous symptoms. The patient sits upright in a chair with a nasogastric tube passed to 30 cm from the nose. Normal saline is infused for 15 minutes followed by 0.1 N HCl for 30 minutes or until symptoms are produced. The test is carried out in such a way that the patient does not know which solution is being perfused. Review of a number of studies reporting this test shows that it has an overall sensitivity of 79% and specificity of 82%[22].

The Bernstein test is useful for assessing patients with atypical pain, particularly in differentiating cardiac from oesophageal pain. If the test is positive, especially if symptoms were evoked early in the acid perfusion, one can be fairly certain that the pain was oesophageal in origin. A negative test does not exclude reflux disease. This test is particularly attractive as it is easy to perform and requires no special equipment.

Acid Reflux Test

A pH probe can be placed in the lower oesophagus and used to detect reflux of gastric acid. To avoid errors this is done in a standard way known as the *Standard Acid Reflux Test*. The pH probe is placed 5 cm from the lower oesophageal sphincter which has been detected manometrically. The pH is then monitored in the basal state and during deep breathing, during Valsalva and Mueller manoeuvres and cough. This is repeated in the right and left decubitus and with the head 20° down. Although this is a simple test in principle it requires specialized equipment and its place is restricted to centres performing oesophageal manometry.

Prolonged Intraluminal pH Monitoring

Recently pH sensitive radiotelemetry capsules have become available for recording the pH of the lower oesophageal lumen for as long as 24 hours while the patient is ambulant. The capsule is swallowed and tethered by a thin polyvinyl tube attached to the cheek with tape[27]. Signals from the capsule are picked up and recorded by a receiver carried by the patient (Figure 2.8). The patient eats a normal diet except that food or drink with a pH of less than pH 5 are avoided. It is possible

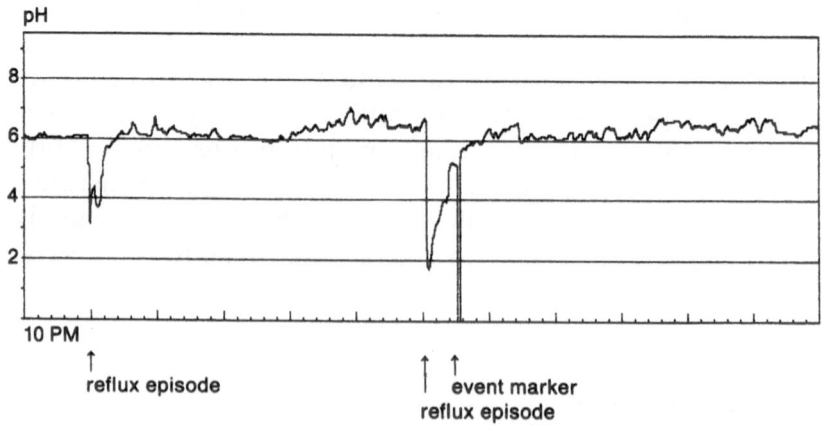

Figure 2.8 Oesophageal pH profile for 1 hour in a patient with reflux disease. There are two reflux episodes but only the second is associated with symptoms as shown by the event marker

to achieve great diagnostic accuracy for reflux with this test with a sensitivity of 88% and a specificity of 98% if the pH is recorded for at least 12 hours[22]. Attempts have been made to make recordings for a shorter length of time but this has reduced diagnostic accuracy.

Intraluminal pH monitoring is the most accurate test available at present for detecting the presence of reflux but it is expensive and requires special expertise. Its place at present is limited to difficult diagnostic problems, perhaps for those patients in whom the result of an acid perfusion test is unclear. It is, however, invaluable for the objective assessment by clinical trial of new therapeutic agents for gastro-oesophageal reflux.

Manometry

Oesophageal manometry requires specialized equipment and expertise and as was discussed earlier, there is no clear correlation between the LOS pressure and reflux, unless many observations are made. It is, therefore, of little value in the diagnosis of reflux disease but may be helpful in selecting the appropriate operation for patients with severe disease. If peristalsis is shown to be poor or absent a tight fundoplication may result in dysphagia and so this operation should be avoided.

Gastrointestinal Scintiscanning

This is an attractive method for the diagnosis of reflux as it avoids the use of tubes. The patient drinks ^{99m}Tc–sulphur colloid in saline which is not absorbed and can be subsequently detected in the upper gastrointestinal tract by gamma camera imaging. Reflux is then provoked by abdominal pressure and postural manoeuvres. Some studies have shown it to be almost as accurate as intraluminal pH monitoring[22]. The radiation exposure is low, less than half of that of a barium meal or a ^{99m}Tc–sulphur colloid liver scan. Its place in the investigation of reflux disease is unclear but it may prove a good screening test in both adults and children.

MEDICAL TREATMENT

The aims of treatment of oesophagitis are to prevent reflux by (1) enhancing the anti-reflux barrier, (2) raising intragastric pH and (3) improving clearance of oesophageal contents by increasing oesophageal peristalsis. All treatments work by one or a combination of these mechanisms.

Physiological Measures

Changes in lifestyle can be very effective in the treatment of oesophagitis and in mild cases are often the only form of treatment required. Some patients find it helpful to eat more regularly, taking their evening meal several hours before going to bed. Benefit is often achieved by avoiding lying down immediately after meals, and if obese by losing weight. Obesity is associated with higher intragastric pressures, which has an unfavourable effect on the LOS and also with impaired clearance of oesophageal contents. The patient is advised to elevate the head of the bed by at least six inches by placing wooden blocks under the legs. It has been shown by continuous intra-oesophageal pH monitoring that this will significantly decrease the number of reflux episodes at night[28].

Diet and Drug Restriction

Some foods such as chocolate, alcohol and carminatives (peppermint, spearmint) have been shown to impair LOS pressure.

Many patients also find that citrus juices, tomato products and coffee are also associated with exacerbation of heartburn. Although they do not have any effect on the LOS pressure they do have a direct irritant action on the inflamed oesophageal mucosa, possibly by an effect related to high osmolarity[29]. Coffee may also alter sphincter pressure and enhance acid secretion in the stomach but at present this is controversial[30].

A number of drugs reduce LOS pressure allowing acid reflux. These drugs include progesterone, theophylline, prostaglandins, all drugs with an anticholinergic action including tricyclic antidepressants and phenothiazines, α-adrenergic antagonists such as phentolamine and dopamine, morphine and calcium-channel blocking drugs such as verapamil and nifedipine. These potentially harmful drugs should be avoided if a suitable alternative is available. Smoking will cause a marked reduction of the LOS pressure, probably because of the anticholinergic effect of nicotine[31]. Patients should be advised to stop smoking tobacco[31].

Antacids

Although antacids have been the mainstay of treatment of oesophagitis there is only scanty evidence of their efficacy from clinical trials. They neutralize the gastric contents and so reduce the acidity of the refluxed material into the oesophagus. They also increase the LOS pressure and decrease reflux[32]. Uncontrolled studies have shown that they are effective in controlling symptoms in 60–70% of patients and also prevent the recurrence of heartburn during the day. One study in 19 patients compared the benefit of continuous intra-oesophageal infusion of a liquid antacid, continuous oesophageal infusion of water, and hourly oral administration of antacids. Both the continuous intra-oesophageal antacid infusion therapy as well as oral antacids significantly improved the patients' response to acid perfusion while reflux symptoms treated with water were unchanged[33]. There are very few data as to whether antacids affect the natural history of oesophagitis, whether they promote healing of oesophagitis and whether they prevent stricture formation. A controlled trial comparing medical therapy with antacids against surgical therapy showed that antacids were able to control symptoms in only 17% of patients for three or more years and were not very effective in patients with severe symptoms, or in those with gross endoscopic oesophagitis and severe sphincter incompetence. However these patients were attending a hospital and so they may have represented a more severe sub-group[34].

Thus, although antacids may be effective in controlling symptoms in patients with mild disease, there is only scanty evidence that they are useful in moderate or severe disease and there is little evidence that they promote healing of oesophagitis. This is perhaps not surprising when one considers that to be effective antacids have to maintain a gastric pH above 4.0 for the full 24 hour period. The maximum number of reflux episodes occur at night when presumably antacids will be least effective. Therefore, antacids when used should be chosen for a high buffering capacity, be in the liquid form and be given at frequent intervals.

Alginate/antacid

Alginate/antacid mixtures react with saliva to form a highly viscous foaming solution which floats on the surface of the gastric pool acting as a mechanical barrier to reflux. The antacid is incorporated into this gel-like layer so that should any reflux occur it will not be acidic. It does not have any effect on the LOS pressure[35]. It has been shown that the number of reflux episodes and the proportion of time with an acidic oesophageal pH were significantly reduced by Gaviscon when compared with placebo[35]. A number of studies have compared Gaviscon to standard antacid therapy and have shown the two forms of treatment to be equally effective in relieving symptoms and improving oesophageal inflammation[36]. Thus although alginate/antacid mixtures are effective in reflux disease they are probably not superior to standard antacid therapy.

H_2-receptor Antagonists

Cimetidine and ranitidine are both H_2-receptor antagonists which inhibit basal and nocturnal acid secretion and that stimulated by food, the vagus and a variety of secretagogues such as gastrin. Therefore, these drugs act in reflux disease by reducing gastric acidity and allowing damaged oesophageal mucosa to heal.

H_2-antagonists have been extensively studied in patients with a wide range of severity of reflux oesophagitis. The majority of trials have demonstrated symptomatic improvement (cimetidine 1.2–1.6/g/d, ranitidine 300–600 mg/d) compared with placebo. Overnight pH monitoring has only been performed in a few studies. In one study patients were treated with cimetidine or placebo and at the same time pH was monitored with an intra-oesophageal pH probe. At six weeks there was a modest reduction in the amount of acid refluxed but there was no significant difference between treatment and placebo group at 12 weeks[40]. Combining the results of 10 trials, it would appear that endoscopic improvement can be expected in 63% of patients treated with cimetidine compared with only 35% of patients receiving placebo[41].

Ranitidine has also been shown to be effective. In one study 36 patients with moderate to severe reflux oesophagitis were randomized to receive either ranitidine 150 mg twice daily or placebo for 6 weeks. There was healing or improvement of endoscopic lesions in 79% of cases treated with ranitidine compared with 24% of those patients receiving placebo. Further benefit was gained in the more resistant cases by continuing the drug for a further 6 weeks[54]. Thus, H_2-antagonists are effective in both relieving symptoms and promoting mucosal healing in patients with all severities of disease. Although there is some evidence that ranitidine is a more potent drug than cimetidine on an equal dose basis, it is not clear if this is clinically important[42]. Other factors such as possible drug interactions and cost should also be considered when choosing which drug to use.

Bethanechol

Bethanechol is a drug which has proved more popular in the USA than in the UK and Europe. It is a cholinergic agent which increases the LOS pressure and enhances oesophageal peristalsis. It has been shown that patients receiving bethanechol 25 mg four times a day had less symptoms and required less antacid than patients taking a placebo[37]. It was also shown to promote the healing of oesophagitis. Overall the results were as good as those from other trials using an H_2-antagonist. However, bethanechol has the disadvantage that gastric secretion is promoted and some patients experience abdominal cramps, diarrhoea, urinary frequency and blurred vision. Nevertheless it may have a useful role in the treatment of oesophagitis particularly if combined with an H_2-receptor antagonist.

Metoclopramide

Metoclopramide is a dopamine antagonist which increases the amplitude of oesophageal contractions and of LOS pressure and stimulates gastric emptying[38]. Unlike bethanechol, it does not affect gastric acid secretion. Clinically, metoclopramide reduces the frequency and severity of heartburn[39]. A disadvantage is the appreciable number of neurological and psychotropic side-effects which occur at the standard dosage, which may limit its use in the treatment of oesophagitis.

Sucralfate

Sucralfate is a new anti-ulcer drug which forms an adherent complex with proteins at site of ulcers forming a barrier against acid, pepsin and bile salts. In one study sucralfate has been compared with standard alginate/antacid therapy. After 6 weeks symptomatic improvement was similar in both groups (69%), as was the extent of healing of oesophageal lesions. Thus sucralfate is at least as effective as alginate/antacids mixtures in the treatment of oesophagitis[55]. Although this drug shows promise it remains to be seen what place it finds in the treatment of oesophagitis.

CONCLUSIONS

The majority of patients can be managed satisfactorily with medical measures alone. Treatment should be undertaken in a stepwise fashion firstly eliminating risk factors such as smoking and optimizing any other drug therapy the patient might be taking. In addition the patient should be advised to raise the head of the bed. If these steps fail to control symptoms then antacids should be given. If treatment at this stage is unsuccessful the patient should be investigated to establish the diagnosis and then given an 8-week course of an H_2-antagonist. If after 8 weeks there is no improvement the H_2-antagonist should be continued for another 8 weeks at a higher dose. Surgery should be considered if there is no substantial improvement after 4 months.

The role of maintenance therapy in reflux oesophagitis once initial healing has been achieved remains controversial. One option is to continue postprandial antacids with a night-time dose of an H_2-antagonist for 3 months. However many patients will require treatment for considerably longer periods of time and some will need it indefinitely to prevent symptomatic relapse. There is one particular group of patients in whom it is difficult to give firm advice. These patients, often elderly, have severe oesophagitis macroscopically and histologically but are symptom-free. There is little evidence that H_2-antagonists prevent stricture formation unless there is mucosal healing. However surgery is difficult to recommend as the patients are frail and asymptomatic. It seems best to manage the stricture, should it occur, by endoscopic dilatation and to try and promote healing of the oesophageal mucosa by medical means.

TREATMENT OF COMPLICATIONS

Strictures

Benign strictures occur most commonly in the elderly who are often unfit for surgery. Fortunately only a minority of these patients will require surgery since most can be adequately treated medically.

Dysphagia, in about one-third of patients, can be treated simply by control of oesophagitis with H_2-antagonists. This is probably because the fibrous component of the stricture is small and reduction of spasm, oedema and restoration of motor function is all that is required[15]. These patients often need maintenance treatment for many years as recurrence of oesophagitis will lead to a return of dysphagia.

Treatment of strictures with intermittent bouginage is now the treatment of choice for most patients as it is effective, generally safe and avoids the need for surgery. A guide-wire is passed through the stricture under direct vision via a fibroptic endoscope. The endoscope is then removed and bougies of the Eder–Puestow or Celestin type are then passed down the guide-wire to dilate the stricture. As many as 40% of patients will require only one dilatation but others will require multiple treatments combined with full medical therapy[43]. Once dilated, most patients do not require more than 2–3 dilatations a year and many patients only have further dilatations 'on demand' as dictated by their dysphagia.

Although intermittent dilatation is far safer than surgery it is not without risk. One study of 1203 patients reported a perforation rate of 0.9% with four deaths, although the perforation rate can be reduced substantially if only experienced endoscopists perform the procedure[44,45].

Surgery should be reserved for the younger patient in whom control with intermittent bouginage is incomplete. As the morbidity and mortality is higher with surgery than bouginage it is not a treatment of first choice and should be strictly reserved for medical treatment failures. Usually an anti-reflux operation is carried out with pre- and post-operative dilatation. Fundoplication is often chosen for short strictures and a Roux-en-Y diversion for long strictures. The mortality associated with resection is high and should be avoided if at all possible.

Barrett's syndrome

Treatment of Barrett's syndrome is traditionally considered to be surgical. The principles of treatment are prevention of reflux, dilatation of associated strictures and resection of adenocarcinomas. Medical treatment is generally ineffective in producing regression of the columnar epithelium. A recent study showed that although the use of antacids and cimetidine over a 1–2 year period does result in symptomatic relief, there was no regression of the columnar epithelium[46]. Early reports of surgical treatment were similar to medical treatment but a more recent study showed regression of columnar epithelium in four of ten patients treated surgically[47]. This correlated with decreased reflux on acid reflux (pH probe) testing.

The majority of carcinomas associated with Barrett's oesophagus will be found at presentation so all suspicious lesions should be biopsied. If a carcinoma-in-situ is found resection should be recommended. However, when dysplasia alone is present it is unclear as to what is the correct course of action. Annual follow-up with endoscopy would seem prudent. It is equally unclear as to what surveillance patients with uncomplicated Barrett's syndrome should be given as the carcinoma detection rate is likely to be low[20]. Again review with endoscopy every 1–2 years would seem sensible.

SURGICAL TREATMENT

About 10% of patients will not be adequately controlled by medical measures and will require surgical intervention. However there are now a bewildering array of possible operations and a marked paucity of well-conducted controlled trials to guide one's choice of procedure. The situation is further complicated as few of the operations are standardized, the term 'Nissen fundoplication' (Figure 2.9) being used to cover a variety of techniques[48].

Before selecting surgical treatment for a patient it should be

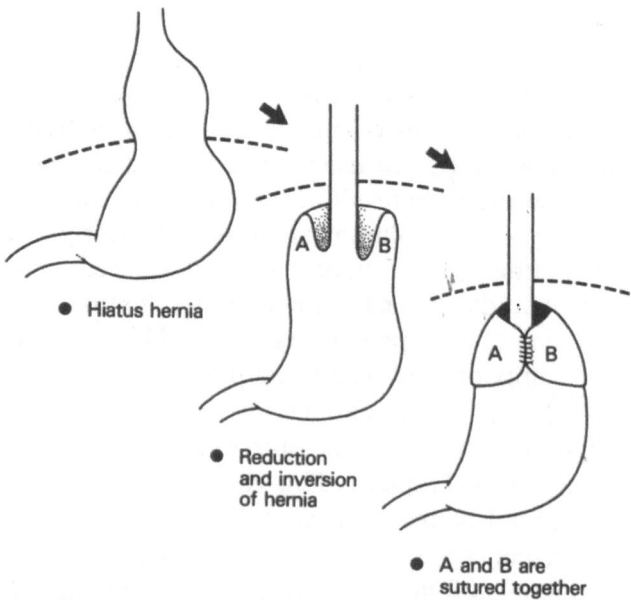

- Hiatus hernia

- Reduction and inversion of hernia

- A and B are sutured together

Figure 2.9   Surgical procedure for Nissen fundoplication for the treatment of hiatus hernia with reflux disease

borne in mind that surgery has a mortality rate of up to 2% in some series which, unless the symptoms are intolerable, is unacceptable for an otherwise benign condition[49]. It therefore behoves the physician to establish with certainty that reflux oesophagitis is present, that the symptoms are caused by the oesophagitis rather than being cardiac or functional and, finally, that adequate medical treatment has been given. Only once these conditions have been fulfilled should the patient be referred for surgery.

The majority of surgeons at present carry out one of the Nissen fundoplication procedures. There is however a significant failure rate ranging from less than 10% to 40%, depending on the definition of failure and the length of follow-up[50]. Moreover in some series up to a third of patients are not satisfied with the results; new symptoms can result from the operation including dysphagia, bloating and inability to vomit and belch ('gas-bloat syndrome')[22]. The corollary of this is that two thirds of patients are helped by surgery when the medical therapy has failed. Nevertheless dissatisfaction with the results of Nissen fundoplication has led to a search for new techniques.

One new approach is the use of a device called an Angelchik prosthesis. This is a doughnut-shaped ring made of silicone plastic filled with silicone gel (Figure 2.10). This is placed around the abdominal oesophagus with tie strap[51]. The advantage is that the surgery is simpler than the Nissen fundoplication and the post-operative morbidity is less. These techniques have recently been studied by a prospective randomized controlled trial. Fifty-two patients were randomized to have either a fundoplication or Angelchik prosthesis. After a 2–4 year follow-up, seven patients in the fundoplication group had poor results whereas reflux was controlled in all the patients with Angelchik prosthesis, though one developed severe dysphagia necessitating removal of the prosthesis. The incidence of the 'gas-bloat' syndrome was far less in the Angelchik patients. There have been reports of serious side-effects such as erosion with perforation of the prosthesis into the

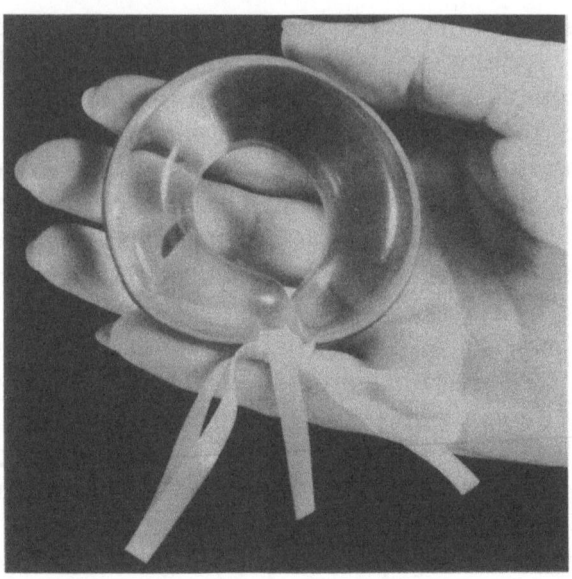

Figure 2.10 Angelchik prosthesis: an alternative to Nissen fundoplication

stomach but these are rare[52]. Further studies are required before its place can be established.

It has been postulated that alkaline reflux is important in the pathogenesis of oesophagitis and this has led to the use of a Roux-en-Y biliary diversion combined with an antrectomy. A prospective randomized controlled trial has tested this technique. 91% of Roux-en-Y patients had good results compared to 65% of patients treated with fundoplication[53]. This difference however was not statistically significant. Again further studies are required before this can be recommended with confidence.

In summary, 10% of patients with oesophagitis will require surgical treatment. Although the majority will be helped by a Nissen fundoplication, a sizeable minority will have unsatisfactory results. The Angelchik prosthesis appears promising and, if further studies confirm the good results obtained to date, this may become the standard procedure in the future.

ACKNOWLEDGEMENTS

The authors gratefully acknowledge financial support by the Wellcome Trust. M.J.G.F. is a Wellcome Trust Senior Lecturer. We are indebted to Drs C. Bartram and A. M. McLean for providing the radiographs shown in Figures 2.5, 2.6 and 2.7, and to Dr I. P. Donlad for supplying the oesophageal pH profile.

REFERENCES

1. Nebel, O. T., Formes, M. F. and Castell, D. O. (1976). Symptomatic gastro-oesophageal reflux: incidence and precipitating factors. *Am. J. Dig. Dis.*, **21**, 953–956
2. Edwards, D. A. W. (1984). Physiology of the oesophagus. In Bouchier, I. A. D., Allan, R. N., Hodgson, H. J. F., Kieghley, M. R. B. (eds.) *Textbook of Gastroenterology*, pp. 18–25. (London: Baillière-Tindall)
3. Dyer, M. H. and Pridie, R. B. (1968). Incidence of hiatus hernia in asymptomatic subjects. *Gut*, **9**, 696–699
4. Dent, J., Dodds, W. J. and Friedman, R. H. (1980). Mechanism of gastro-oesophageal reflux in recumbent asymptomatic human subjects. *J. Clin. Invest*, **65**, 256–267.
5. Dodds, W. J., Dent, J. and Hogan, W. J. (1978). Pregnancy and the lower oesophageal sphincter. *Gastroenterology*, **74**, 1334–1335
6. Van Thiel, D. H., Gavalier, J. S. and Stremple, J. F. (1979). Lower oesophageal sphincter pressure during the normal menstrual cycle. *Am. J. Obstet. Gynecol.*, **134**, 64–67
7. Demish, G. W. and Castell, D. O. (1971). Inhibitory effect of smoking on the lower oesophageal sphincter. *N. Eng. J. Med.*, **284**, 1136–1137.
8. Nebel, O. T. and Castell, D. O. (1972). Lower oesophageal sphincter changes after food ingestion. *Gastroenterology*, **63**, 778–783
9. Cohen, S., Fisher, R. and Lipschutz, W. (1972). The pathogenesis of oesophageal dysfunction in sclerodema and Raynaud's Disease. *J. Clin. Invest.*, **51**, 2663–2668
10. Vantrappen, G. and Hellemans, J. (1980). Treatment of achalasia and related disorders. *Gastroenterology*, **79**, 144–154
11. Chung, R. S., Johnson, G. M. and Den Besten, L. (1977). Effect of sodium taurocholate and ethanol on hydrogen ion absorption in rabbit oesophagus. *Am. J. Dig. Dis.*, **22**, 582–588
12. Hamon, J. W., Johnson, L. F. and Maydonovitch, C. L. (1981). Effects of acid bile salts on the rabbit oesophageal mucosa. *Dig. Dis. Sci.*, **26**, 65–72
13. Booth, D. J., Kemmerer, W. D. and Skinner, D. B. (1968). Acid clearing from the distal oesophagus. *Arch. Surg.*, **76**, 732–734

14. Orr, W. C., Johnson, L. F. and Robinson, M. G. (1984). Effects of sleep on swallowing, esophageal peristalsis and acid clearance. *Gastroenterology*, **86**, 814–819
15. Bennett, J. R. (1984). Oesophagitis. In Bouchier, I. A. D., Allan, R. W., Hodgson, H. J. F. ,and Kieghley, M. R. B. (eds.) *Textbook of Gastroenterology*. pp. 40–50. (London: Baillière-Tindall)
16. McCallum, R. W., Berkowitz, D. M. and Lewar, E. (1981). Gastric emptying in patients with gastroesophageal reflux. *Gastroenterology*, **80**, 285–291
17. Bennett, J. R. (1983). Chest pain – heart or gullet? *Br. Med. J.*, **286**, 1231–1232
18. Barrett, N. R. (1957). The lower oesophagus lined by columnar epithelium. *Surgery*, **41**, 881–894
19. Sarr, M. G., Hamilton, S. R., Marrone, G. C. and Cameron, J. L. (1985). Barrett's oesophagus: its prevalence and association with adenocarcinoma in patients with symptoms of gastroesophageal reflux. *Am. J. Surg.*, **149**, 187–193
20. Cameron, A. J. C., Orr, B. J. and Payne, W. S. (1985). The incidence of adenocarcinoma in columnar-lineal (Barrett's) esophagus. *N. Engl. J. Med.*, **313**, 857–859
21. Cohen, S. and Harris, L. D. (1971). Does hiatus hernia affect competence of the gastroesophageal sphincter? *N. Engl. J. Med.*, **284**, 1053–1056
22. Richter, J. E. and Castell, D. O. (1982). Gastroesophageal Reflux: Pathogenesis, Diagnosis and Therapy. *Ann. Intern. Med.*, **97**, 93–103
23. Ott, D. J., Wu, W. C. and Gelford, D. W. (1981). Reflux esophagitis revisited: prospective analysis of radiographic accuracy. *Gastroint. Radiol.*, **6**, 1–7
24. Ismail-Beigi, F., Horton, P. F. and Pope, C. E. (1970). Histological consequences of gastroesophageal reflux in man. *Gastroenterology*, **58**, 163–174
25. Ismail-Beigi, F. and Pope, C. E. (1974). Distribution of the histological changes of gastroesophageal reflux in the distal oesophagus of man. *Gastroenterology*, **66**,1109–1113
26. Knuff, T. E., Benjamin, S. B., Worsham, G. F., Hancock, J. E. and Castell, D. O. (1984). Histologic evaluation of chronic gastroesophageal reflux. An evaluation of biopsy methods and diagnostic criteria. *Dig. Dis. Sci.*, **29**, 194–201
27. Branicki, F. J., Evans, D. F., Ogilvie, A. L., Atkinson, M. and Hardcastle, J. D. (1982). Ambulatory monitoring of oesophageal pH in reflux oesophagitis using a portable radiotelemetry system. *Gut*, **23**, 992–998
28. Johnson, L. F. and Demeester, T. R. (1981). Evaluation of elevation of the head of the bed, bethanechol and antacid foam tablets on gastroesophageal reflux. *Dig. Dis. Sci.*, **26**, 673–680
29. Lloyd, D. A. and Borda, I. T. (1978). Food-induced heartburn: effect of osmolarity. *Gastroenterology*, **75**, 240–243
30. Thomas, K. B., Stembaugh, J. T., Fromkes, J. J., Mekhjian, H. S. and Callwell, J. H. (1980). Inhibitory effect of coffee on lower esophageal sphincter pressure. *Gastroenterology*, **79**, 1262–1266

31. Demmish, G. W. and Castell, D. O. (1971). Inhibitory effect of smoking on the lower esophageal sphincter. *N. Engl. J. Med.*, **284**, 1136–1137
32. Castell, D. O. and Levine, S. M. (1971). Lower oesophageal sphincter response to alkalinization. A new mechanism for treatment of heartburn with antacids. *Ann. Intern. Med.*, **74**, 223–227
33. Serebro, H. A., Friedman, M. and Beck, I. T. (1973). Efficacy of continuous intra-oesophageal antacid drip therapy in the treatment of reflux oesophagitis. *South Afr. Med. J.*, **47**, 1656–1659
34. Behar, J., Sheaham, D. G., Biancani, P., Spiro, H. M. and Storer, E. H. (1975). Medical and surgical management of reflux oesophagitis. *N. Engl. J. Med.*, **293**, 263–268
35. Stanciui, C. and Bennett, J. R. (1974). Alginate/antacid in the reduction of gastro-oesophageal reflux. *Lancet*, 109–111
36. Graham, D. Y., Lanza, F. and Dorsch, E. R. (1977). Symptomatic reflux oesophagitis: a double-blind controlled comparison of antacids and alginate. *Curr. Ther. Res.*, **22**, 653–658
37. Farrell, R. L., Roling, G. T. and Castell, D. O. (1974). Cholinergic therapy of chronic heartburn. *Ann. Intern. Med.*, **8**, 573–576
38. Stanciu, C. and Bennett, J. R. (1973). Metoclopramide in gastroesophageal reflux. *Gut*, **14**, 275–279
39. McCallum, R. W., Ippoliti, A. F., Cooney, C. and Sturdevant, R. A. L. (1977). A controlled trial of metoclopramide in symptomatic gastroesophageal reflux. *N. Engl. J. Med.*, **296**, 354–357
40. Bennett, J. R., Martin, H. D. and Buckton, G. (1980). Cimetidine in reflux oesophagitis. In: Hepato-Gastroenterology Supplement. *Abstracts of the XI. International Congress of Gastroenterology.* June 8–13, Hamburg, p. 30.
41. Tytgat, G. N. J. (1981). Assessment of the efficacy of cimetidine and other drugs in oesophageal reflux disease. In Baron, J. H. (ed.) *Cimetidine in the 80's.* pp. 153–166. (Edinburgh: Churchill Livingstone)
42. Mahachai, V., Walker, K. and Thomson, A. B. R. (1985). Comparison of cimetidine and ranitidine on 24-hour intragastric acidity and serum gastrin profile in patients with esophagitis. *Dig. Dis. Sci.*, **30**, 321–328
43. Watson, A. (1984). The role of antireflux surgery combined with fibreoptic endoscopic dilatation in peptic esophageal stricture. *Am. J. Surg.*, **148**, 346–349
44. Dawson, J. and Cochel, R. (1981). Oesophageal perforation at fibreoptic gastroscopy. *Br. Med. J.*, **1**, 283–285
45. Lee, M., Ravenscroft, M. M., Green, J. R. B. and Swan, C. H. J. (1983). Safe outpatient dilatation of benign oesophageal strictures. *Gut*, **24**, A1008
46. Wesdorp, I. C. E., Bartelsman, J., Schipper, M. E. I. and Tytgat, G. N. (1981). Effect of long-term treatment with cimetidine and antacids in Barrett's oesophagus. *Gut*, **22**, 724–727
47. Brand, D. L., Ylvisakes, J. T., Gelfand, M. and Pope, C. E. (1980). Regression of columnar esophageal (Barrett's) epithelium after antireflux surgery. *N. Engl. J. Med.*, **302**, 844–848

48. Jamieson, G. G. and Duranceau, A. (1984). What is a Nissen fundo-
    plication? *Surg. Gynaecol. Obstet.*, **159**, 591–596
49. Polk, H. C. (1976). Fundoplication for reflux esophagitis. *Ann. Surg.*,
    183, 645–682
50. Gear, M. L. W. (1985). In Jewell, D. P. and Chapman, R. W. (eds.)
    Topics in Gastroenterology. pp. 135–145. (Oxford: Blackwell Scientific
    Publications)
51. Angelchik, J. P. and Cohen, R. (1979). A new surgical procedure for the
    treatment of gastroesophageal reflux and hiatal hernia. *Surg. Gynaecol.
    Obstet.*, **148**, 246–248
52. Pickleman, J. (1983). Disruption and migration of an Angelchik eso-
    phageal anti-reflux prosthesis. *Surgery*, **93**, 467
53. Washer, G. F., Gear, M. W. L., Dowling, B. L., Gillison, E. W.,
    Royston, C. M. S. and Spencer, J. (1984). Randomized prospective trial
    of Roux-en-Y duodenal diversion versus fundoplication for severe reflux
    esophagitis. *Br. J. Surg.*, **71**, 181
54. Wesdorp, I. C. E., Dekker, W. and Klinkenberg-Knol, E. C. (1983).
    Treatment of reflux oesophagitis with ranitidine. *Gut*, **24**, 921–924
55. Laitinen, S., Stahlberg, M., Kairaluoma, M., Kivinienn, H., Paakkonen,
    M., Lahtinen, J., Poikolainen, E. and Ankee, S. (1985). Sucralfate and
    alginate/antacid in reflux esophagitis. *Scand. J. Gastroenterol.*, **20**, 229–
    232

3

PEPTIC ULCER

M. LANCASTER-SMITH

INTRODUCTION

The epidemiological profiles of gastric and duodenal ulcer have changed considerably during the twentieth century and herein may lie valuable clues to their aetiologies.

Both are diseases with a worldwide distribution and it has been estimated that 10% of Western society experience peptic ulceration. It is, therefore, not surprising that requests to investigate patients considered to have peptic ulcer constitute approximately 40% of referrals to gastrointestinal departments in the United Kingdom. However only in one half of these will an ulcer be confirmed, which perhaps indicates that our traditional diagnostic data base requires reappraisal or refinement.

Although the burgeoning of endoscopy services has undoubtedly extended our understanding of the nature of peptic ulcer, it has also led in many instances to over-enthusiastic and inappropriate monitoring of dyspepsia and a devaluation of clinical assessment.

The healing of peptic ulcer is, in the vast majority of cases, no longer a problem with the advent of modern drugs and the promise of even more potent agents. Prevention of relapse remains the main therapeutic challenge and although drugs also have a role in this area the place of surgery is being reappraised, because it offers a potentially permanent cure.

These particular topics are addressed in this chapter. The clinical diagnosis of dyspepsia is discussed in more detail in Chapter 4 and the pathogenesis of peptic disease is the subject or Chapter 1. Complications of peptic disease and their management are largely omitted because in the main these are the province of hospital-based services.

CLINICAL FEATURES

The clinical features of peptic ulcer and other causes of dyspepsia are more fully discussed in Chapter 4. The following summary is largely derived from the work of Crean and his colleagues[1] at the Southern General Hospital, Glasgow and other recent analyses of gastrointestinal symptoms by De Dombal[2] and Lennard Jones[3].

The characteristic symptom of peptic ulcer is epigastric pain – *indeed the absence of epigastric pain makes peptic ulcer an exceedingly unlikely diagnosis.* But epigastric pain is also a prominent feature of many other digestive system diseases and is therefore of little discriminatory value.

By contrast the grouping of symptoms in individual patients can be used to discriminate with considerable accuracy. The following features characterize peptic ulcer and those disorders from which it should be distinguished.

(1) *Peptic Ulcer*

   (a) Frequent nocturnal pain relieved by food, milk or antacid

   (b) History longer than four years

   (c) Bouts of pain more frequent in winter

(d) Patient feels like taking food soon after vomiting

(e) Points with finger to epigastrium when asked to identify site of pain

(2) *Gastric Carcinoma*

(a) Patient over 50 years old

(b) Short history of dyspepsia

(c) Daily pain

(d) Weight loss

(e) Early fullness with meals

(3) *Alcohol-related Dyspepsia*

(a) Male

(b) Admission of high alcohol intake

(c) Nausea and retching before breakfast

(d) Painless diarrhoea

(e) Little abdominal pain

(4) *Non-organic Dyspepsia including the Irritable Bowel Syndrome*

(a) Poorly localized pain which is infrequently nocturnal

(b) Disturbed bowel function

(c) Pellet stools and incomplete rectal emptying

(d) Relief from pain with defaecation or passing flatus

Crean has extended this approach and adapted it for computer interrogation and analysis. The system has been evalu-
ated in a primary health care setting with considerable success
and acceptability from both practitioners and patients. Hopefully, it will be effective in improving diagnostic decision making in dyspepsia and reduce the cost of investigation and

treatment. If so it will deserve more widespread application in health centres.

DEFINITIONS

Sites

The overwhelming majority of peptic ulcers occur in the duodenum and stomach. Of all duodenal ulcers 90% occur within the first part of that organ. The lesser curve and in particular the incisura remains the commonest site of gastric ulceration. Although the aetiologies of gastric and duodenal ulcer are probably distinct the two disorders may coexist.

Ulcers are less frequently found in the oesophagus usually as a complication of gastro-oesophageal reflux (see Chapter 2), and even more rarely at the anastomosis of gastric and intestinal mucosa following gastric surgery. In the rare Zollinger–Ellison syndrome the jejunum may ulcerate as may the ileal mucosa adjacent to ectopic gastric mucosa in a Meckel's diverticulum.

Erosions and Acute Ulcers

Erosions are best defined as breaks in the mucosa that do not penetrate the muscularis mucosa. They are usually no larger than 2–3 mm in diameter, multiple and most frequently found in the gastric fundus. They are associated with traumatic stress, shock, septicaemia, hepatic and renal failure, severe burns and non-steroidal anti-inflammatory drugs (NSAID). Healing is usually complete within 1–2 weeks and scarring does not occur.

A small proportion of such lesions fail to heal rapidly forming acute ulcers which penetrate deeply leading to perforation and clinically identifiable haemorrhage.

Although the pathogenesis of these acute lesions may be similar to the early stages of chronic ulceration the two conditions appear to be distinct. However in the case of NSAID-induced damage it seems that long-term usage may produce lesions that are not easily distinguished from 'spontaneous' chronic ulcers.

Chronic Ulcer

Chronic peptic ulcers penetrate through the muscularis mucosa and are characterized by fibrotic scarring and deformity.

EPIDEMIOLOGY

The main aim of epidemiology is to identify the rates of disease within populations, communities and sub-groups in the hope of identifying causative factors. Unfortunately the true peptic ulcer rate is not accurately known principally because there are no universally accepted clinical criteria for diagnosis. Endoscopy and double contrast radiology are accurate identifying techniques but both are clearly unsuitable for screening large asymptomatic populations. Furthermore, numerical assessment is made difficult by the remitting and relapsing nature of the disease and the fact that symptoms of an ulcer and its presence do not always coincide.

The main sources of epidemiological information on peptic ulcer are:

(1) *Mortality Statistics*
Because peptic ulcer rarely causes death, mortality rates are of very limited value in measuring the prevalence of the disease within a community.

(2) *Autopsy Findings*
Signs of active or previous chronic ulceration at post-mortem examination gives unequivocal evidence of the disease, but it is likely that subjects coming to autopsy

are a selected and unrepresentative sub-group of the general population under study.

(3) *Hospital Admission and Out-patient Referral Rates*
The frequency of referral for peptic ulcer to hospitals with a well-defined catchment area that has a stable population provides valuable information. Nevertheless the accuracy is affected by variations in the criteria used for referral by general practitioners and the declared special interests and skills of hospital consultants.

Admission rates for bleeding and perforation are unlikely to be influenced by such factors and have been used to compare present with past incidence rates and one region with another. A valid criticism of this technique is that complications occur in only a minority of cases and it may therefore be unreasonable to draw conclusions about the total spectrum of the disease from this information. In particular the natural history of a disease frequently changes with time and so too may its complication rate.

(4) *Population Surveys*
Survey of a defined population is the most accurate measure of incidence and prevalence. In the past clinical assessment and confirmation by barium meal have been used. Endoscopic monitoring would be even more accurate but for practical and ethical reasons the survey would have to be restricted to dyspeptic individuals. This would undoubtedly underestimate the frequency of ulcer disease because ulcers are not always symptomatic.

Definitions

Point Prevalence

The frequency of the disease in a defined population at a fixed point in time.

Period Prevalence

The frequency of the disease in a defined population during a specified period e.g. a year or a life-time.

The Incidence

The number of new cases occurring during a given time in a specified unit of population, e.g. number of new cases per year per 1,000 population.

Incidence and Prevalence

Both duodenal and gastric ulcer are worldwide diseases. In a population survey conducted in London by Doll and his colleagues[4] the prevalence of peptic ulcer varied from 1.8% of the total population aged under 25 years to 9.6% in the 45–55 age group. Using necropsy data Watkinson[5] found a similar age related rise in prevalence with frequencies of 0.5% in those under 25 and a maximum of 7.1% in the 55–65 age group. More recently Ihamaki, Varis and Siurala[6] using endoscopy found a point prevalence in an adult Finnish population of 1.68% for active peptic ulcer. Studies from America suggest that the minimum life-time prevalence for peptic ulcer is approximately 10%. In Western Europe duodenal ulcer is four to five times more common than gastric ulcer[6,7].

The incidence of new duodenal ulcer cases reported by Pulvertaft[7] in York was 0.215% for men and 0.062% for women. For gastric ulcer the figures were 0.053% and 0.031% for men and women respectively. More recent reports from Denmark by Bonnevie[8,9] reveal comparable figures of 0.18% and 0.08% for duodenal ulcer and 0.05% and 0.04% for gastric ulcer in men and women respectively. An even more recent similarly designed study in the USA[10] demonstrated a considerably lower frequency than the Danish data. For duodenal ulcer the incidence was approximately 50% lower than in Denmark and for gastric ulcer approximately 30% below the Danish level. The reasons for these lower American frequencies are not clear but possibly indicate that the American population studied was not representative of the USA in general because the National Centre for Health Statistics[11] found a significantly higher peptic ulcer incidence of 0.29% in 1975.

Assuming that these data are applicable to the United Kingdom it can be estimated that *there are approximately 80 000 new cases of peptic ulcer each year and that during a 12 month period about one million of the population suffer from the condition.*

Effect of Age and Sex on Peptic Ulcer Incidence

In the nineteenth century peptic ulcer was found most commonly in the stomachs of young women[12]. However, during the early part of this century in the United Kingdom the frequency of the disease in men rose with duodenal ulcer becoming 10–20 times and gastric ulcer 4–8 times commoner in men than women. Since the early 1950's the male to female ratio for gastric ulcer has changed very little in Western Europe, whereas there has been a significant reduction in the

Table 3.1   Ulcer in the United Kingdom and Scandinavia. Mean annual incidence rates per 1000 population aged 15 and over

		Gastric ulcer		Duodenal ulcer	
		Men	Women	Men	Women
York, England	1952–57	0.5	0.3	2.2	0.6
SW Scotland	1957–59	0.4	0.3	5.4	1.3
Rogaland, Norway	1950–52	0.6	0.3	2.4	0.6
Copenhagen County	1963–68	0.5	0.4	1.8	0.8

ratio for duodenal ulcer (Table 3.1) which now stands at approximately 2:1[9]. This is strictly comparable to more recent data from the USA[10].

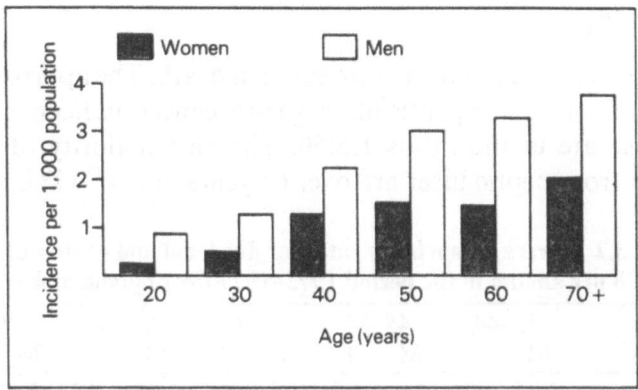

Figure 3.1 Incidence of duodenal ulcer per 1000 population in Copenhagen, 1963–68

For duodenal and gastric ulcer the incidence increases with age in both men and women as exemplified by Danish figures[8,9], (see Figures 3.1 and 3.2) and confirmed by Kurata and colleagues in the USA[10].

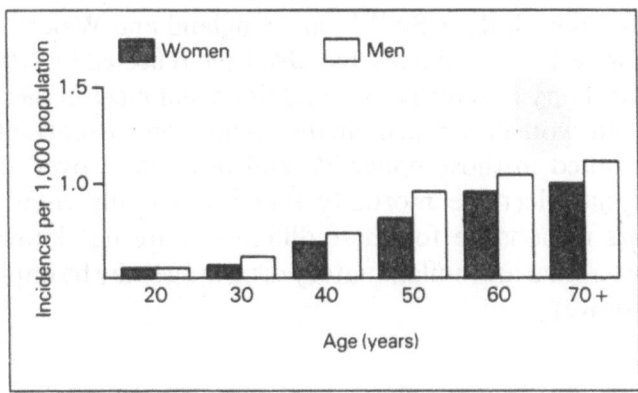

Figure 3.2 Incidence of gastric ulcer per 1000 population in Copenhagen, 1963–68 (from Lancaster-Smith (1983). *Peptic Ulcer*. London: Update Publications)

Mortality

Peptic ulcer is a relatively rare cause of death. The approximate mortality rates for peptic ulcer, gastric cancer, ischaemic heart disease are in the ratios 1:5:50. The vast majority of those dying from peptic ulcer are over 65 years of age[13] (Table 3.2).

Table 3.2   Average mortality rates for duodenal and gastric ulcer per 100 000 per annum in the period 1973–1977 for England and Wales

Age	35–44		45–54		55–64		65–74		75+	
Sex	M	F	M	F	M	F	M	F	M	F
DU	0.95	0.21	3.4	1.2	8.5	2.4	23.5	6.8	58.6	24.0
GU	0.56	0.30	2.2	1.0	7.2	3.1	20.2	10.0	57.3	41.6

From reference 13
M – Male; F – Female

Changing Pattern of Peptic Ulcer

In the nineteenth century gastric ulcer was infinitely more common than duodenal ulcer[12]. During the first 50 years of this century the prevalence of duodenal ulcer steadily rose. However since the 1950's there appears to have been a steady decline in the incidence of peptic ulcer, especially for duodenal disease in both the USA[14–17], and England and Wales[13,18].

This declining incidence has also been reflected in a decreasing mortality rate for gastric and duodenal ulcer in men of all ages. In women a much smaller reduction in mortality has been noted in those under 75, and in patients over 75 with duodenal ulcer the mortality rate has actually risen[13]. The factors responsible for these differences are not known but non-steroidal anti-inflammatory drug usage may be implicated (see above).

Seasonal Patterns

There is a widely held opinion that peptic ulcer occurs and recurs most frequently in the spring and autumn. However,

Kurata and Haile[19] on reviewing relevant literature published between 1925 and 1982 were unable to identify any consistent pattern although there is probably a trend for ulcers to cause death or bleed during summer months.

Geographical Differences

Based on regional admission rates for peptic ulcer the prevalence of duodenal ulcer appears to be higher in the North of England than the South and to be greater still in Scotland

Table 3.3 Regional UK admission rates of men with peptic ulcer per 1000 population in 1967

	Duodenal ulcer	Gastric ulcer
East Anglia	0.84	0.54
Wessex	0.89	0.39
Liverpool	1.59	0.47
Newcastle	2.26	0.59
Scotland	2.94	0.57

(Table 3.3). By contrast gastric ulcer shows little geographical variation in the United Kingdom.

In certain areas of India the DU:GU ratio is as high as 30:1. There is an apparent prevalence rate 20 times greater in Southern India compared to the North[20]. This is a far wider regional variation than can be found in Western Europe and North America.

International comparison of absolute incidence and prevalence rates is largely invalid because of widely varying standards and methods of recording, diagnosing and managing peptic disease.

Social Class

Mortality figures from the first quarter of this century suggest that gastric ulcer was a disease most prevalent in semiskilled and unskilled workers but that duodenal ulcer was commoner amongst professional and managerial sections of society. In contrast more recent data from Britain and the USA show that both gastric and duodenal ulcer increase in prevalence with decreasing social class and educational achievement[21].

ENVIRONMENTAL FACTORS

The changing pattern of peptic ulcer during the past 100 years surely suggests that environmental factors must be implicated in the aetiology of the disease. Yet evidence for this hypothesis is far from conclusive for most of the suggested factors.

Smoking

Smokers[22] and those with a previous history of smoking[23] have an increased risk of developing peptic ulcers.

Furthermore the frequency of peptic ulceration increases with the number of cigarettes smoked[24]. The association between smoking and ulcer is stronger for men than for women[25,26].

Healing of peptic ulcer is delayed[27-29] and the relapse rate increased by continuing to smoke[30]. Smoking appears to decrease healing rates even in those taking H_2 antagonists perhaps by reducing the inhibition of gastric secretion achievable with these drugs.

The pathogenetic relationship between smoking and peptic ulcer is not clear. In gastric ulcer there may be a relationship to the decrease in pyloric sphincter tone induced by nicotine[31,32] which in turn encourages gastroduodenal reflux (Chapter 1). In addition nicotine reduces pancreatic bicarbonate secretion[33] which would inevitably diminish neutralization of gastric acid in the duodenum and possibly predispose to ulceration. It also has been proposed recently that smoking interferes with the output of prostaglandin E_2[34] which is considered to be important in protecting the upper gastrointestinal tract.

Alcohol

There is no clear evidence that alcohol causes or exacerbates peptic ulcer[23,26,35]. Duodenal ulcer occurs more frequently in patients with cirrhosis but this is probably due to the liver dysfunction rather than the alcohol per se[36].

Diet

Coffee – stimulates gastric acid secretion[37] and previous heavy consumption of coffee has been linked to the later development of duodenal ulcer[23]. However a strong direct association between the two could not be confirmed[26,38].

As with coffee, *Cola-type* soft drinks may be associated with the subsequent development of duodenal ulcer[23].

So called 'gastric' diets do not enhance healing[39–41]. By contrast, diets requiring mastication may be protection[42] and high fibre regimes seem to reduce the rate of duodenal ulcer recurrence[43].

Drugs

Aspirin – Regular users of aspirin, especially women, have an increased incidence of gastric ulcer[35,44,45]. The mechanism is not certain but aspirin is known to allow damaging back diffusion of hydrogen ions into the gastric mucosa[46] and to inhibit the synthesis of cytoprotective prostaglandins[47].

Corticosteroids – High or prolonged dosage of corticosteroids undoubtedly predisposes to or exacerbates peptic ulcer[48] but it is also possible that even in moderate doses steroids may be implicated in causing ulcers of the stomach and duodenum[49].

Non-steroidal anti-inflammatory drugs (NSAID) – These drugs induce acute ulcers in the upper gastrointestinal tract of experimental animals probably by interfering with prostaglandin synthesis. It is not clear whether they induce chronic ulceration in man but there is now considerable evidence to suggest that they are responsible for the increasing incidence or peptic ulcer haemorrhage[50] and perforation[51,52] in the elderly.

Apart from ibuprofen, which seems to be the least toxic of the NSAID group, there is no evidence that any one drug is less toxic than the others.

Psychological Factors

Although changes in the gastric mucosa[53] and increased secretion[54] are known to occur under stress, the evidence that stressful life events cause or exacerbate peptic ulcer is mostly negative[55,56,57]. Weiner *et al.*[58] following a prospective psychological analysis successfully predicted the subsequent development of peptic ulcer in a group of military recruits, but apart from this study there is no sound evidence to support the concept of an 'ulcer personality'.

Genetic Factors

The possible genetic basis of peptic ulcer has recently been reviewed[59]. In summary:

(1) siblings of patients with gastric or duodenal ulcer have approximately 2.5 times the incidence of these diseases compared to controls, but there is no hereditary link between the two diseases.

(2) the possession of blood group O or the absence of blood group antigens in mucosal secretions is associated with a small increased incidence of duodenal ulcer[60].

(3) the presence of hyperpepsinogenaemia is accompanied by an increased incidence of duodenal ulcer.

How these factors influence peptic ulceration is not clear,

Relief of Pain

Recent carefully controlled studies have shown either no significant relief[61] or only a slight improvement[62,63] of ulcer pain after a single dose of antacid compared with placebo. Against this are the many decades of apparent user satisfaction declared by those who took antacids on a *regular* basis for their ulcer, prior to the introduction of carbenoxolone and H_2 antagonists.

Healing

Only in the past 10 years have antacids been shown to enhance the healing of peptic ulcers. Peterson and colleagues[64] showed that a combination of magnesium and aluminium hydroxides in very large doses (210 ml per day) with a neutralizing capacity greater than 1000 mEq accelerates duodenal ulcer healing comparable to cimetidine. The amounts of antacid involved and the looseness of stool caused by the regime make it unacceptable for routine use but subsequent trials have found that regimes with approximately 200–300 mEq neutralizing capacity per day enhanced ulcer healing[65,66].

Prevention of Relapse

Almost 30 years ago Cayer *et al.*[67] showed that compared to placebo, antacid tablets taken four times daily (2 hours after meals and at bedtime) reduced the rate of recurrence and return of symptoms in peptic ulcer patients over an 8 month study period.

The major advantage of antacid therapy is the comparative lack of serious unwanted effects and relative inexpensiveness. Nevertheless they are not entirely free of problems.

Sodium bicarbonate should not be used on a long-term

basis because it is readily absorbed and may cause significant alkalosis.

Aluminium salts often constipate, possibly by interfering with bile salt metabolism.

Other rarer clinical problems due to chronic ingestion include.

(1) Phosphorus depletion[68]

(2) Fluoride malabsorption[69]

(3) Reduced absorption of drugs (tetracyclines, iron, prednisolone, H_2 antagonists)

(4) Aluminium toxicity syndrome in patients with renal failure.

Magnesium salts – the major and often limiting unwanted effect is diarrhoea probably caused by the osmotic purgative effect of insoluble magnesium salts in the lumen of the intestine or by decreasing transit time due to the release of cholecystokinin.

The combination of aluminium and magnesium salts in many proprietary preparations largely overcomes the disturbance that the individual salts have on bowel function.

Calcium-containing compounds rapidly neutralize hydrochloric acid but should be avoided because calcium stimulates gastrin release and leads to rebound hypersecretion of acid[70]. Chronic use of calcium carbonate may also cause hypercalcuria and nephrocalcinosis.

It should be remembered that the multitude of antacid preparations on the market have widely varying buffering capacities[71] (Table 3.4).

Antimuscarinic Anticholinergic Drugs

Drugs in this category imitate the actions of atropine, the most important of which are:

(1) To decrease bronchial, salivary secretion and gastric secretion

(2) To decrease sweating

(3) Dilatation of the pupils and inhibition of accommodation

(4) To increase heart rate

(5) Inhibition of micturition and intestinal motility.

Atropine is efficiently absorbed from the alimentary tract but it also readily crosses the blood–brain barrier giving rise

Table 3.4 The buffering capacities of proprietary antacids. From reference 71

Antacid	Neutralizing capacity (ml of 0.1 N HCl) per 10 ml of antacid or per tablet
Liquids	
Magnesium trisilicate BPC	220
Aluminium hydroxide gel BPC	255
Antasil	428
Maalox	233
Polycrol gel forte	230
Mylanta	220
Asilone gel	194
Asilone suspension	301
Mucaine	294
Liquid Gaviscon	55
Tablets	
Magnesium trisilicate BPC	45
Aludrox	142
Antasil	204
Maalox	240
Polycrol forte	100
Asilone	105
Gaviscon	15
Nulacin	93
Gelusil	65
Actal	84

to unpleasant central effects. By contrast the so-called atropine like drugs, most of which are quaternary ammonium compounds (e.g. propantheline, poldine, glycopyrronium, benzilonium) are poorly and erratically absorbed especially when taken with food[72,73]. The main advantages that these drugs have over atropine are the relative lack of central side effects due to poor transfer across the blood–brain barrier and the comparatively small blocking effect at ganglionic level.

There seems little doubt that when these drugs are given intravenously or in large oral doses gastric secretion of acid and pepsin is significantly reduced, however their effectiveness after oral administration of ordinary doses has been questioned[74,75].

These obvious defects in specificity and erratic absorption led to the search for an efficiently absorbed drug with selective antimuscarinic action on gastric secretion. Such claims have been made and partially substantiated for *pirenzipine*[76–78].

Healing and Symptom Relief

Until the advent of pirenzipine there were few acceptable studies demonstrating a healing effect of anticholinergic drugs in peptic ulcer. This is mainly because the majority of such drugs were introduced before endoscopic monitoring was available. Recently propantheline thrice daily and at night was shown to be equivalent to cimetidine 1 g daily in healing duodenal and pyloric ulcers[79]. Similar comparability with cimetidine has been demonstrated in duodenal ulcer patients for combinations of antacids and 1-hyoscyamine[80] and propantheline[81].

Between 1979 and 1982 large numbers of trials were published showing that pirenzipine 100–150 mg daily accelerates the healing of peptic ulcer compared to placebo and gives comparable results to cimetidine and ranitidine for healing and symptom relief. Lower doses of pirenzipine are less effective than H_2 antagonists. These results are fully reviewed by

Walan[82]. Side effects at this dosage were not uncommon, the most frequent being dry mouth in 13.5% and visual disturbance in 6.3%[78].

Prevention of recurrence

Many of the older antimuscarinic drugs used on a long-term basis appear to reduce the complication and recurrence rate of duodenal ulcer[82]. Pirenzipine 100 mg daily reduces the relapse rate compared to placebo[83] but is probably less effective than cimetidine 400 mg daily.

H_2 Antagonists

Histamine has long been considered the most important final mediator of parietal cell stimulation. However conventional antihistamines (H_1 antagonists) have no significant action on gastric secretion and it was therefore postulated that there are different histamine receptors on parietal cells. We now know these as H_2 receptors.

Two drugs which selectively block these receptors are clinically available in the United Kingdom, cimetidine and ranitidine. Both drugs reduce gastric secretion and inhibit stimulation by histamine, pentagastrin, the vagus or food[84,85].

Healing and Symptom Relief

Cimetidine There is overwhelming evidence from a large number of trials throughout the world published between 1976 and 1982 that cimetidine rapidly relieves symptoms in the great majority of patients with duodenal ulcer and that healing is accelerated[86]. A minority of trials have shown no significant difference in the rate of healing achieved with cimetidine compared with placebo which seems to be largely explicable on the basis of very high placebo healing rates in some parts of the world[87,88]. Approximately 80% of duodenal ulcers will heal in 4–6 weeks compared with an average placebo healing rate of 40%. After 8–12 weeks on cimetidine more than 90% will have healed[89]. There seems to be no appreciable difference between the dosage regimes of 200 mg t.d.s. and 400 mg nocte or 400 mg b.d., however 800 mg nocte may confer additional healing power[90]. Cimetidine also relieves symptoms in gastric ulcer and healing rates after 4–12 weeks therapy may be comparable to those in duodenal ulcer[91,92].

Ranitidine   Ranitidine has been available since 1981 compared with cimetidine which has been on the UK Market since 1976.

To date all published trials have demonstrated a superiority over placebo[86]. The average healing rate on ranitidine has been 80% compared to 30% for placebo after a 4–6 week treatment period.

In gastric ulcer also symptom relief and healing comparable to that with cimetidine have been found[93,94]. The dosage regime most commonly used has been 150 mg b.d. but 300 mg nocte may be even more effective, at least in duodenal ulcer[95].

Ranitidine 300 mg daily and cimetidine 1 g daily appear to be equally effective in *healing* duodenal ulcer when compared directly in the same trial[86]. Nevertheless duodenal ulcers failing to heal on conventional doses of cimetidine appear to be responsive in many instances to ranitidine[96,97].

If H_2-blocking drugs are given for 12 weeks more than 90% healing can be achieved[98], even so a small proportion of duodenal ulcers are resistant to these drugs which may be due to a failure of H_2 antagonists sufficiently to reduce nocturnal gastric secretion in some patients[99].

Prevention of recurrence

That peptic ulcer is a relapsing disease has been particularly emphasized in recent years by the very high recurrence rates found in endoscopically monitored long-term maintenance trials of H_2 antagonists. These studies have also shown that recurrence of ulceration seen endoscopically is considerably more common than symptomatic relapse[89,98]. Furthermore, prolonging the full dose healing course of an H_2 antagonist for up to 2 years does not reduce the relapse rate after the drug has been stopped, which remains at approximately 8.5% per month[89].

Numerous trials have shown that cimetidine 400 mg nocte and ranitidine 150 mg nocte effectively reduce the relapse rate of duodenal ulcer compared with placebo[86]. For cimetidine the rate of recurrence is approximately 2.5% per month against recurrence on placebo of 8.5%[89]. A recent large multi-centre trial which directly compared the efficacy of cimetidine 400 mg nocte and ranitidine 150 mg nocte in duodenal ulcer show a significantly lower relapse rate in patients taking ranitidine over a 12 month period[100].

Even so H_2 receptor blocking drugs do not eliminate recurrence. This partly is due to poor compliance but it seems likely that in some patients low dose H_2 blockade is insufficient to maintain the healed state.

Gastric ulcer is also notorious for its high recurrence rate after healing[101]. Both cimetidine[102,103] and ranitidine[104] significantly reduce this relapse rate.

Unwanted Effects of H_2 Antagonists

Cimetidine Considering that many millions of patients have taken cimetidine over the past decade reports of adverse effects are extremely rare.

The most important are:

(1) Drowsiness and confusion, especially in the elderly and those with renal or hepatic impairment. Dosages should therefore be reduced to at least half of those normally recommended in the 65-plus age group

(2) Gynaecomastia and impotence due to antiandrenogenic activity

(3) Very rare cholestasis in children and rather more commonly mild elevation of hepatic transaminases which are reversible and considered to be insignificant

(4) Inhibition of the hepatic cytochrome P450 enzyme system which therefore increases the blood concentration of drugs metabolized by this pathway – these include, anticoagulants, anticonvulsants, diazepam and propranolol.

Ranitidine　Reports of unwanted effects with ranitidine are even more uncommon. It does not have any significant effect on the cytochrome P450 system or antiandrogenic activity.

Carcinogenicity　Because achlorhydria and hypochlorhydria in pernicious anaemia and after gastrectomy are associated with an increased incidence of gastric malignancy[105,106] suspicion has been raised about the dangers of gastric antisecretory drugs. It has been suggested that low levels of gastric acidity allow the proliferation of bacteria that are capable of producing from food nitroso-compounds which are potentially carcinogenic[107]. It has also been proposed that H_2 antagonists could be metabolized to carcinogens in the gastric lumen, but this has not been substantiated by *in vivo* studies nor have experimental animals on these drugs developed malignant stomach lesions[108,109]. Furthermore in an extensive post-marketing surveillance study of cimetidine *no causal link was found between the drug and gastric carcinoma*[110]. It therefore seems highly likely that anecdotal reports of gastric cancer in patients on cimetidine[111,112] are no more than chance occurrences. Nevertheless practitioners should be alert to the possibility that H_2 antagonists may mask the symptoms of cancer and may allow partial healing of malignant lesions[113].

In conclusion it can be said that both cimetidine and ranitidine are very safe drugs. Ranitidine has a cleaner profile and should be used whenever there is a possibility of drug interaction. Ranitidine is considerably more expensive and seems to be no more effective than cimetidine in *healing* the majority of duodenal or gastric ulcers. For long-term prevention of relapse ranitidine appears to have the advantage.

New Antisecretory Drugs

Famotidine

Famotidine is a new and potent H_2 receptor antagonist which is likely to be released in the United Kingdom in the near future. In man it is 40–60 times more potent than cimetidine and 12–15 times more potent than ranitidine and has a longer duration of action than both of these drugs. Early studies show that it is comparable to cimetidine and ranitidine in healing and preventing relapse of peptic ulcers. It is apparently safe and free of major adverse effects.

Omeprazole

Omeprazole is a substituted benzimidazol that inhibits secretion of gastric acid by interfering with the action of the enzyme H^+-K^+-ATPase. It is long-lasting and is a potent antisecretory drug. More than 90% of duodenal ulcers heal in 2–4 weeks with omeprazole 20 mg–60 mg daily and the vast majority are asymptomatic within seven days[114,115]. The relapse rate on stopping the drug is comparable to that found after H_2 receptor antagonist treatment[115]. Its exact role in the treatment of peptic disease has yet to be established.

Sucralfate

Sucralfate is a basic aluminium salt of sucroseoctasulphate. In an acid environment (pH < 4) some aluminium ions dissociate from the octasulphate molecules which polymerize, forming a viscous paste. In this form sucralfate binds preferentially to denatured protein in the ulcer base forming a protective layer[116,117]. The mechanism of action probably includes:

(1) Protection of the ulcer from further 'acid attack'

(2) Reduction of peptic activity

(3) Adsorption of bile salts[116,118,119,120].

Healing and Symptom Relief

In two large placebo controlled trials sucralfate enhanced the healing of duodenal ulcer, with rates of 75–80% at 4–6 weeks[121,122]. Furthermore healing rates and symptom relief in duodenal ulcer with sucralfate are comparable to cimetidine[123].

The most common dose regime has been 1 g four times daily but 2 g twice daily seems to be equally effective[124].

Sucralfate and cimetidine are equally efficacious in the healing of gastric ulcer[125,126].

Prevention of Relapse

Maintenance treatment with sucralfate 1–3 g daily significantly reduces the relapse rates of duodenal ulcer[127,128] and gastric ulcer[129]. For both diseases the relapse rates whilst taking sucralfate are very similar to those achieved with H_2 receptor antagonists.

Unwanted Effects

The overall incidence of side-effects is very low with constipation being the most commonly reported. Nausea, dry mouth and diarrhoea have also been noted. Although very little aluminium is absorbed from sucralfate, there is a theoretical risk of toxicity in patients with renal failure.

Bismuth

Tripotassium dicitratobismuthate in a colloidal alkalinated solution (Denol) was originally only available in liquid form, but is now marketed as a chewable tablet. Colloidal bismuth chelates with the proteins in the base of an ulcer forming a protective layer. Hydrogen ions are prevented from reaching the ulcer base[130] and the colloidal bismuth layer also binds pepsin and bile salts[131]. It has no significant antacid action but does suppress gastric pepsin secretion[170]. Colloidal bismuth requires an acid medium to be active and is therefore most effective when taken one hour before meals and at bedtime.

Healing and Symptom Relief

Numerous placebo controlled trials have demonstrated the efficacy of colloidal bismuth in gastric[132–134] and duodenal ulcer[123], with healing rates up to 96% after 4–6 weeks treatment. Strictly comparable promotion of healing to cimetidine has also been shown[123].

Prevention of Relapse

Continuous long-term usage of bismuth compounds has not been adopted because of fears about possible neurotoxicity. These are probably unfounded because blood levels of bismuth rise only slightly during routine use and are well below the accepted safety limit. Nevertheless the usual recommendation is to allow two months between healing courses of the drug. There is evidence[135,136] though not universal[137] that ulcers healed with colloidal bismuth remain healed longer than those healed by H_2 receptor antagonists. Why this should be so is not known.

Other Drugs

Carbenoxolone

Although it undoubtedly promotes the healing of peptic ulcers it can no longer be recommended now that alternative preparations are available, because of its sodium retaining and potassium losing properties.

Deglycyrrhinnized liquorice (Caved S and Ulcedal)

These appear to have some healing effect in peptic ulcer but are not comparable to the previously discussed drugs.

Trimipramine (Surmontil)

This enhances the healing of peptic ulcers, though the mechanism is not clear. Rates of healing tend not to be as impressive as those achieved with H_2 antagonists[123]. Side effects include drowsiness and dry mouth.

Prostaglandin analogues

Prostaglandins are a group of naturally occurring cyclic fatty acids which have a very wide range of activity. One group inhibits gastric secretion and has an intrinsic mucosal protective action. Synthetic analogues have been produced and are soon to be promoted for the healing of peptic ulcer. Their efficacy is probably dependent upon:

(1) Stimulating protective mucus and bicarbonate secretion

(2) Increasing mucosal blood flow

(3) Stimulating mucosal repair

(4) Inhibiting gastric secretion.

These substances enhance the healing of peptic ulcers but are probably less effective than cimetidine or ranitidine[138-140]. Perhaps their most logical use will be prophylactic, especially in patients taking non-steroidal anti-inflammatory drugs.

MANAGEMENT POLICIES

The Initial Approach

The discriminatory clinical features of peptic disease are fully discussed in Chapter 4.

Clearly it is unnecessary and impractical to investigate every patient who has symptoms compatible with peptic ulcer. So when, on clinical grounds, peptic ulcer seems likely in a patient *under 40 years of age*, it is reasonable to give a single course of ulcer healing treatment combined with general advice which should include the following points:

(1) Take three *normal* meals per day – 'gastric' diets do not enhance healing[39] but increasing dietary fibre may prolong remissions[43]

(2) Stop smoking – there is increasing evidence that smoking is an important factor in ulcer relapse[141]

(3) Alcohol up to two units daily will not delay healing and may be allowed

(4) Excessive coffee consumption should be avoided

(5) Avoid prolonged use of aspirin and NSAI drugs.

Many patients will achieve good results with this approach and providing attacks are infrequent subsequent episodes may be dealt with in similar fashion. All such patients nevertheless must be warned that peptic ulcer is generally a recurrent problem for which as yet there is no definitive medical cure. If symptoms recur rapidly and frequently or are not adequately relieved, investigation to confirm the diagnosis and exclude alternative pathologies is appropriate. Furthermore if dyspepsia occurs for the first time in a patient *over 40 years* old investigation should preferably precede treatment with ulcer healing drugs to prevent confusion and delay in diagnosing possible gastric cancer.

The Role of Radiology and Endoscopy

The choice between radiology and endoscopy in the investigation of suspected peptic disease is largely dependent upon what services are available locally. Barium meal is still the most commonly requested investigation by general practitioners but as endoscopic services become more freely available 'on demand' the situation is likely to change.

Accuracy

Duodenal Ulcer   A single contrast barium meal may miss between 20–30% of duodenal ulcers demonstrable by a foreward viewing fibre optic endoscope[142,143]. Double contrast studies appear to be more accurate, because they allow closer examination of the mucosa, missing only 11–20% of endoscopically detected duodenal ulcers[144]. Endoscopy in expert hands is capable of detecting more than 90% of duodenal ulcers[145]. Nevertheless the technique is not perfect and duodenal ulcers not found with the endoscope may sometimes be visualized by X-ray[146]. Scarring from recurrent ulceration and previous surgery make accurate radiological assessment extremely difficult and in these circumstances endoscopy is the investigation of choice. Duodenitis is also likely to be missed on barium meal whereas this important feature is readily seen with the gastroduodenoscope.

Gastric Ulcer   Cotton and Shorvon[147] reviewing a decade of reports comparing endoscopy and radiology in the diagnosis of gastric ulcer found substantial agreement between the two techniques. Nevertheless, disagreement does occur and in many studies endoscopy was just as likely to miss ulcers as a double contrast barium meal. Many radiologists claim to be able to distinguish with a high degree of accuracy benign from malignant gastric ulcers, but endoscopy has the major advantage in this context because multiple biopsies can be obtained at both the initial and follow-up examination. Theoretically this should make diagnosis of malignancy certain, but it seems not to be the case and approximately 5% of malignant lesions may still be missed even when this protocol is adopted[148].

More subtle lesions of the stomach such as gastritis and dysplasia are not easily detected by radiology and, therefore, endoscopy has a clear advantage in these diagnostic categories.

Safety   Barium meal examination has an extremely low morbidity and a virtually nil mortality rate. The dose of irradiation is small and is only significant when young patients require repeated studies. It is of course also inappropriate for pregnant women. Endoscopy, performed usually under sedation with intravenous diazepam, is also very safe. Nevertheless complications such as cardiorespiratory depression and perforation of the oesophagus do happen and death attributed to the procedure occurs once every 5000–10 000 examinations[149]. Endoscopy may transmit infection, viral hepatitis and Salmonella being notable examples, and barium meal is therefore preferable in patients known to be infected.

Choice of Investigation   For many general practitioners wishing to investigate a dyspeptic patient there is no choice because as yet upper gastrointestinal endoscopy is not universally available 'on demand'. When it is, I believe endoscopy should be requested as the initial investigation because it has the greater potential definitive diagnostic yield. The possible exception to this is if the presenting complaint is true dysphagia (obstructed swallowing), when many endoscopists are unhappy to proceed until a barium swallow has been done. If a barium meal is chosen and shows duodenal ulcer there is no indication to perform an additional endoscopy. Even if the radiologist is able only to demonstrate scarring and deformity of the duodenal bulb and the patient's symptoms are compatible with active ulceration there is *no* need to request endoscopy, because management is unlikely to be affected.

When a gastric ulcer is found on barium studies and the radiologist believes the lesion is benign the patient should be given a healing drug and endoscopy arranged for 6 weeks later to check that healing is complete and that the radiologist's estimation of non-malignancy is correct. If the radiologist is uncertain endoscopy should be undertaken before treatment to allay fears and avoid delay in the diagnosis of possible malignancy. If an initial endoscopy and histological examination show the lesion is 'benign', follow-up endoscopy should still be arranged after 6 weeks treatment because mistakes do occur[148]. Even so there is sadly no evidence that open access endoscopy for dyspeptic patients improves the survival rate from gastric cancer in the United Kingdom[150].

The Long-term Problem

Despite recent advances in drug therapy peptic ulcer remains a long-term problem for the majority of patients. It is impossible to be dogmatic about the choice of a regimen because this will vary greatly from one patient to another. The following are possible management approaches:

(1) Certainly many patients, possibly the majority, keep themselves free of symptoms by the occasional very short-term use of antacids or other more potent healing drugs and the efficacy of this approach has been validated[151]

(2) Others, with long asymptomatic remissions will happily take a full dose 6 week course of an ulcer healing drug whenever symptoms return. Probably more than two-thirds of patients with duodenal ulcer can be managed in this way[152,153]

(3) A third group, usually because of the severity of their disease may reasonably be selected for low dose maintenance therapy after the initial full dose healing course[89]. Severity in this context is difficult to define, but the criteria include:

(a) A bleed on more than one occasion

(b) A penetrating ulcer

(c) An average of more than three relapses per year (the cost of four 6-week healing courses of an H_2 receptor antagonist is roughly equivalent to that of a single healing course and 46 weeks low dose maintenance).

In addition the old and those suffering from other diseases, who might be embarrassed by a complication of their ulcer, should also seriously be considered for maintenance therapy.

The length of long-term treatment is impossible to define because the course of the disease varies widely from one patient to another. Fry[154] studying patients with peptic ulcer who in the main did not require hospital referral and therefore presumably had relatively mild disease, found that 90% were asymptomatic or little troubled by their disease 10 years after diagnosis. Symptoms in this group reached a peak during the seventh year after onset. In contrast patients referred to hospital, who are therefore likely to have more severe disease, appear to have a less favourable prognosis. Scandinavian studies on such groups[155,156] have shown in duodenal ulcer that within 13 years more than 20% had undergone surgery and that in those followed for 18–33 years 43% had received an operation. At the same stages of follow-up only 37% and 20%

respectively were asymptomatic. Gastric ulcer appears to have a comparable long-term prognosis. At 18–33 years after diagnosis 32% had required surgery, 15% had continued to experience severe symptoms and only 29% were asymptomatic.

In summary therefore 'long-term treatment' is likely to be at least 7 years and possibly much longer in many patients. *There are no clinical or investigational markers to assist the decision when to stop maintenance treatment* and all that can be advised is occasional trial withdrawal of the drug to see whether treatment is still needed.

Ulcers Resistant to Healing

Duodenal Ulcer

Approximately 20% of duodenal ulcers remain unhealed after a 4–6 week course of H_2 receptor antagonist, sucralfate or Denol although the proportion that remain symptomatic is smaller. If the healing course is extended to 12 weeks less than 10% are resistant[98]. Nevertheless, a small number of duodenal ulcers remain problematical despite prolonging treatment with the initially chosen drug. A number of alternative regimes have been tried and available evidence indicates that:

(1) Ulcers not healing with cimetidine may do so with ranitidine[157] or Denol[158]

(2) The combination of cimetidine and pirenzipine is no better for healing resistant ulcers than continuing with cimetidine alone[159]

(3) The main indication for omeprazole, when available, may be for the healing of ulcers resistant to other drugs, because of its very potent antisecretory action[160]

(4) Surgery remains a viable alternative treatment for duodenal ulcers resistant to drug therapy[161].

Gastric Ulcer

As with duodenal ulcer true resistance to drug therapy is rare. Gastric ulcers are usually larger than duodenal ulcers and not surprisingly take longer to heal. Therefore 3 months continuous full dose treatment is often necessary to complete healing. Failure to heal may be an indication that the radiologist, endoscopist and histologist were wrong in their initial assessment that the lesion was benign. Further endoscopic and histological review is therefore *obligatory* when healing is incomplete after 3 months treatment. Providing malignancy has been excluded and the patient's symptoms are controlled it is reasonable to continue medical management for a further 3 months. If the lesion remains unhealed despite this extension of therapy and the patient is a good operative risk surgery should then be seriously considered.

Treatment failure in peptic ulcer should also pose the following questions:

(1) Has the patient stopped smoking? There is now growing evidence that smoking seriously impairs the healing of peptic ulcer, especially duodenal lesions[141]

(2) Is he or she taking non-steroidal anti-inflammatory drugs?

(3) Are the ulcer healing drugs being taken as prescribed?

(4) Could the patient have the Zollinger–Ellison syndrome?

Ulcers that Keep Relapsing

As discussed true resistance to healing is very rare in peptic ulcer. By contrast relapse on stopping treatment is eventually almost inevitable. Although this can be significantly reduced by prophylactic therapy, recurrence is by no means eliminated. The pattern of relapse varies enormously from one patient to another and a dogmatic regimen cannot be adopted. The

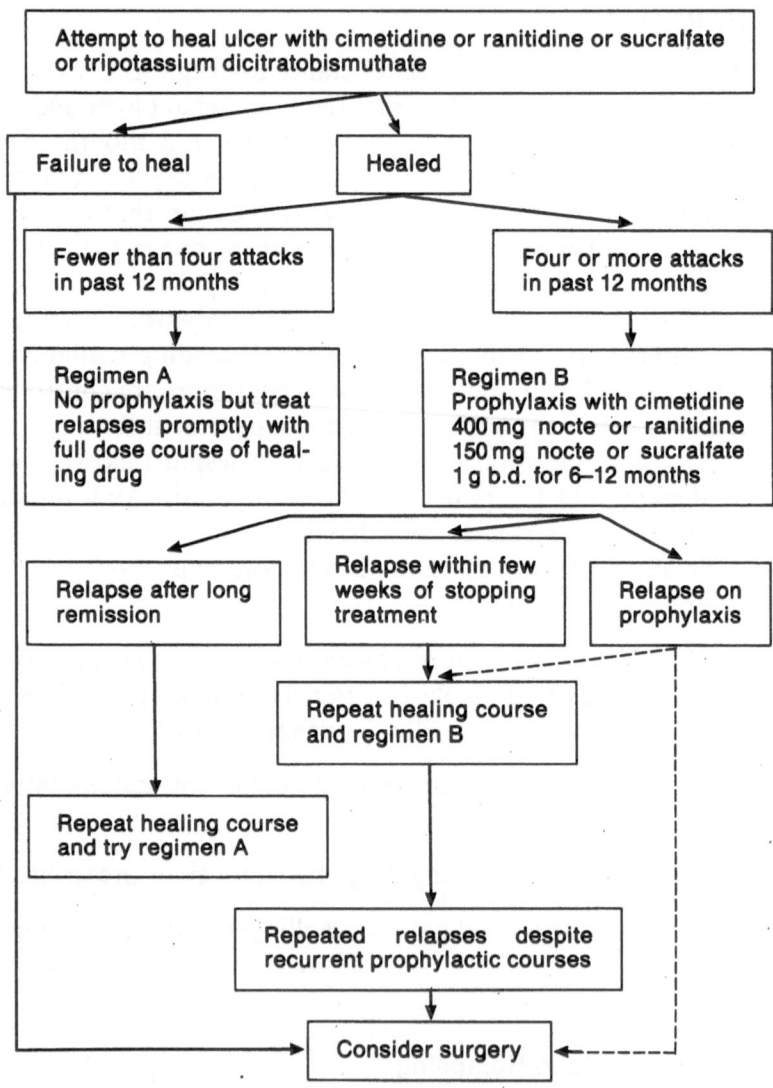

N.B. For patients with *duodenal ulcer* progress may be monitored clinically and follow-up endoscopy or radiology is unnecessary in the great
majority of patients. *Gastric ulcer* healing, whenever possible, should be
checked endoscopically. If healing is incomplete rebiopsy should be
performed to ensure that the lesion is benign.

Figure 3.3 Suggested   Regimens of Management for Uncomplicated Peptic Ulcer

scheme illustrated in Figure 3.3 is therefore offered only as a guide. Decisions regarding long-term policy will need to consider:

(1) The patient's preference for medical or surgical management

(2) Frequency of relapse or development of ulcer complications

(3) Potential operative risk, e.g. does the patient have additional cardiorespiratory disease?

(4) Age – it would seem entirely reasonable to offer drug prophylaxis to elderly patients with uncomplicated ulcer rather than refer them for surgery

(5) Local surgical skills.

Long-term Endoscopic Follow-up

Because both gastric and duodenal ulcers almost invariably relapse it is reasonable to assume that return of the *same* symptoms, in a patient previously shown to have peptic ulcer, is due to recurrence. Repeated endoscopy is unlikely to provide useful additional information and is therefore unnecessary in the great majority of patients. It should be reserved for:

(1) Complications such as bleeding or pyloric stenosis

(2) *New* symptoms such as anorexia, weight loss or dysphagia, which could indicate additional malignant pathology

(3) Treatment failure, especially when referral to a surgeon is being contemplated

(4) Return of symptoms after ulcer healing surgery.

The Role of Surgery

In the majority of patients, surgery, in contrast to medical treatment, provides a cure for gastric and duodenal ulcer. Despite this the number of operations for peptic ulcer has been steadily declining[162]. This reduction has undoubtedly been accelerated by the introduction of cimetidine in 1975 but other likely reasons are the falling incidence of ulcer disease and the acceptance by physicians and surgeons that a significant proportion of patients are dissatisfied with the result of their operation.

All operations for peptic ulcer aim to reduce gastric acid secretion. This can be achieved by resection of a variable portion of the stomach or section of the vagus nerve. The most commonly performed operations are illustrated in Figures 3.4–3.7.

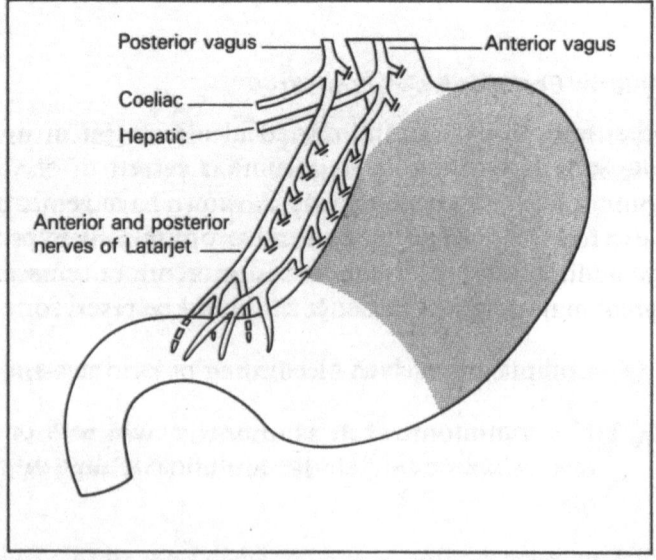

Figure 3.4 Proximal gastric vagotomy. This technique of highly selective vagotomy leaves the motility of the antrum and pylorus unaffected, so that a drainage procedure is not required

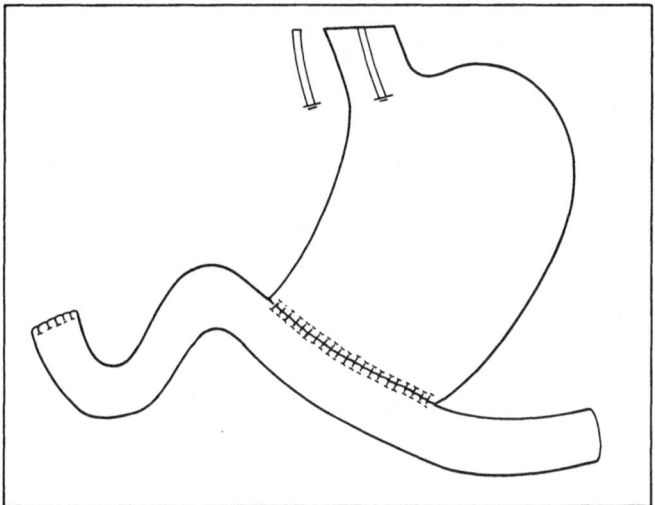

Figure 3.5 Vagotomy and anterectomy aims to reduce acid secretion by removing both gastrin-secreting tissue and the neural stimulation of the parietal cells

Duodenal Ulcer

The exact proportion of patients with duodenal ulcer requiring surgery is not known but is at present probably less than 10%. Failure of medical management accounts for approximately 50% of patients coming to operation. Within this group are those who:

(1) Continue to have severe symptoms from an ulcer that fails to heal after extended courses of ulcer healing drugs

(2) Repeated relapse within a few weeks of stopping a healing course of treatment, particularly if they are unhappy to accept maintenance treatment

(3) Frequently relapse whilst on a maintenance regimen

(4) Have a long history of frequent severe exacerbations and do not wish to persist with medical therapy.

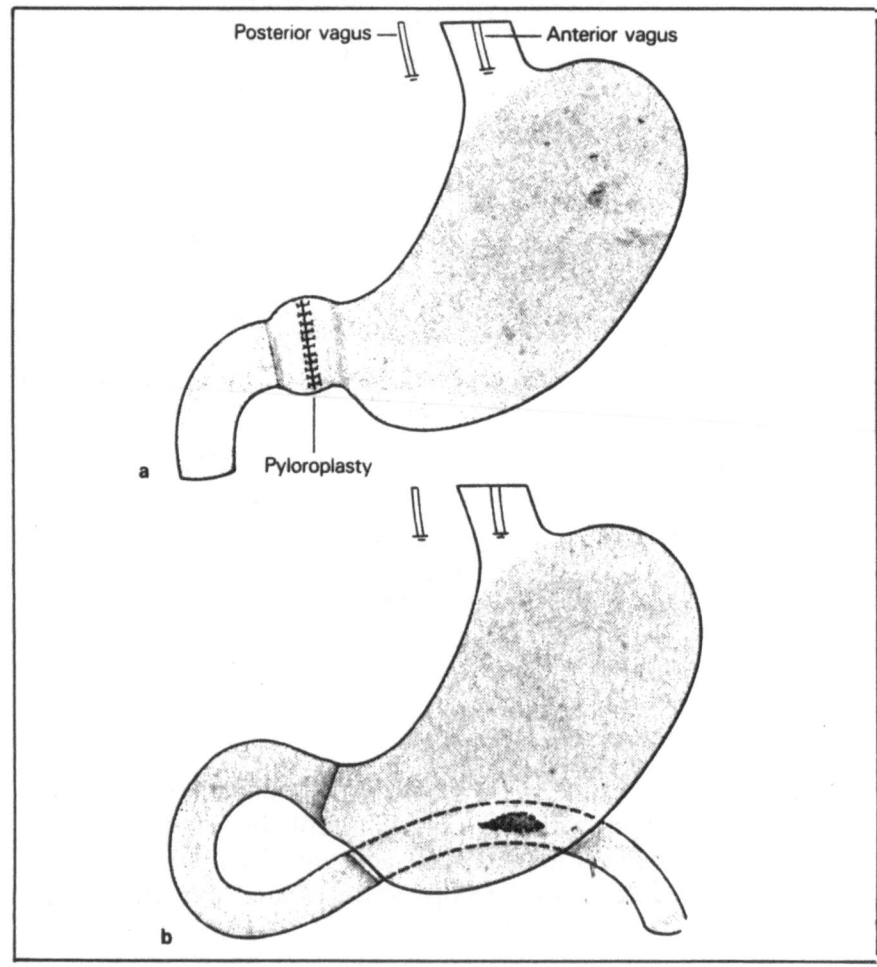

Figure 3.6 Truncal vagotomy leads to gastric stasis and so is combined with a drainage procedure, most commonly pyloroplasty (a). In the presence of duodenal scarring and deformity, however, a gastrojejunostomy (b) is less hazardous.

Other factors that favour surgical referral are a past history of bleeding, particularly if this has occurred more than once, and previous perforation. The remaining 50% of patients receiving definitive surgery have their operation because of

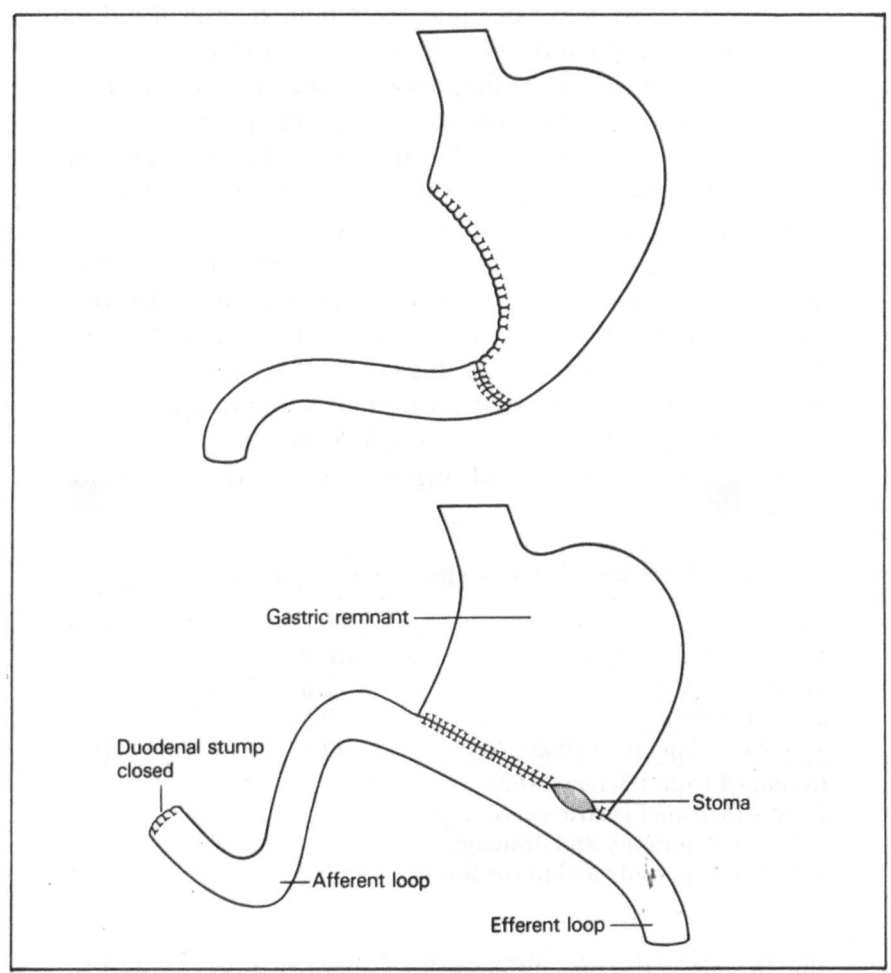

Figure 3.7   In partial gastrectomy approximately two-thirds of the distal stomach is resected. The remnant is then anastomosed either (a) to the duodenum (Bilroth I gastrectomy) or (b) to the jejunum (Bilroth II gastrectomy).

acute complications such as haemorrhage, pyloric stenosis or perforation.

Selection of operation   The over-riding consideration in deciding on which operation must be its mortality rate. However an operation with a low mortality is of limited value if it does not cure the presenting disease or leaves the patient with symptoms that are worse than those of the ulcer itself. These include recurrent ulceration, diarrhoea, dumping, vomiting, gastric stasis and nutritional disturbance. It must also be remembered that if a second operation is necessary this will inevitably increase the overall mortality.

Global assessment   Global assessment and patient satisfaction are difficult to measure but Visick grading is probably the best means of attempting this. A comparison of proximal gastric vagotomy, vagotomy with drainage and vagotomy combined with antrectomy shows that no particular operation is more successful than another[163]. Approximately 20–30% are dissatisfied with the outcome of surgery although the reasons for

Table 3.5   Incidence of adverse effects following gastric surgery

	PGV	V & D	V & A
Ulcer recurrence (%)	10–20	8	1
Diarrhoea (%)	2.6	8.3	2
Dumping (%)	2.8	10.7	22
Visick grading dissatisfied (%)	22	29	18

(modified from reference 162)
PGV = Proximal gastric vagotomy
V & D = Vagotomy and drainage
V & A = Vagotomy and antrectomy

the dissatisfaction are different for each operation (Table 3.5).
Mortality   Operative mortality for gastrectomy, though lowered in recent years by improved anaesthetic and post-operative care, remains at 1–2%. By contrast vagotomy and drainage has a mortality only one tenth of this figure and proximal gastric vagotomy in some series has been achieved without fatalities[164].

Recurrent ulcer rates   Cumulative data from Europe and the USA show that recurrence of ulcer after proximal gastric vagotomy is 10–20%; following vagotomy and drainage it is approximately 8%, whereas the rate after vagotomy and antrectomy is only one per cent[163] (Table 3.5). Bilroth I gastrectomy for duodenal ulcer is associated with an unacceptably high recurrence rate but by contrast after Polya gastrectomy the recurrence rate is only 2%.

Diarrhoea and Dumping   The rates for persistent or recurrent diarrhoea and dumping after various types of surgery are shown in Table 3.5. These problems occur in reverse proportion to the ulcer recurrence rate.

Other problems such as *bilious vomiting* and *gastric stasis* are also considerably less common after proximal gastric vagotomy than the other operations. *Iron deficiency* anaemia occurs in up to 50% and *vitamin B12 deficiency* in 2% after partial gastrectomy but neither appear to be a complication of proximal gastric vagotomy or vagotomy and pyloroplasty.

Treatment of Post-Surgical Recurrent Ulcer   The majority of recurrent ulcers after surgery for duodenal ulcer heal successfully with H_2 receptor antagonists and remain under control with prophylactic therapy[165]. Surgery for recurrent ulcer need only be considered if medical treatment fails to control symptoms and there seems little doubt that vagotomy and antrectomy is then indicated[166].

Other post-surgical syndromes will decrease with the reduction in the numbers of gastrectomies and truncal vagotomies now being performed.

The management of the common problems are summarized below:

Diarrhoea   – codeine phosphate and/or loperamide
Dumping   – small low carbohydrate, high fat meals with no added liquid; post-prandial recumbency; guar additives to delay gastric emptying
                – reversal of the previous drainage procedure
Iron deficiency – annual haemoglobin on all patients with gastrectomy *or* life long low dose prophylactic oral iron.

Gastric Ulcer

The indications for surgery in gastric ulcer are the same as those for duodenal ulcer, namely failure of medical management and occurrence of complications. In practice the operation is frequently offered earlier than in duodenal ulcer because complete healing is more difficult to achieve and complications such as bleeding and perforation have a worse prognosis which mainly reflects the older age of many gastric ulcer patients. Furthermore even when multiple biopsies show no evidence of cancer there is always the suspicion that a persisting gastric ulcer may be malignant.

Selection of operation   Until recently the selection of the operation for gastric ulcer was less controversial than for duodenal ulcer. This is because more than 80% of those treated by the traditional *Bilroth I* procedure are satisfied with the result, the mortality is only 1% and the recurrence rate after long-term follow-up is low at 1–5%[167]. Another reason for favouring gastrectomy is that the actual ulcer is excised thus ensuring that a 'missed' malignant ulcer will not be left. Nevertheless 15–20% of patients having a Bilroth I gastrectomy will be dissatisfied with the result and for this reason alternative operations have been proposed.

Vagotomy and drainage with local resection of the ulcer has been compared with gastrectomy[168] but it appears to be no safer and the recurrent ulcer rate is somewhat higher. *Proximal gastric vagotomy* and local resection to the ulcer has been advocated as a safer alternative to gastrectomy. Adverse sequelae occur less often but ulcer recurrence in most series is higher than normally expected after gastrectomy[161,167].

Pyloric and prepyloric ulcers are considered to be similar in pathogenesis and behaviour to duodenal ulcers and for this reason some form of vagotomy is often performed. The addition of a drainage procedure in this group appears to confer additional benefit[169].

The adverse sequelae of surgery for gastric ulcer are the

same as those after duodenal ulcer operations and their management is based upon the same principles.

In conclusion, although the great majority of patients with duodenal or gastric ulcer can be managed successfully with modern drug therapy, some will prefer surgery either because drugs have failed or because surgery offers a potentially permanent cure. Surgery has become more attractive in recent years due to the advent of proximal gastric vagotomy with its extremely low incidence of adverse sequelae. Even though some patients suffer from recurrent ulceration after this procedure the great majority can be managed with drug therapy and thus avoid a potentially risky second operation.

REFERENCES

1. Crean, G. P. (1984). Symptomatic diagnosis of dyspepsia. In Lancaster Smith, M. J. (ed.) *Peptic Ulcer*, pp. 14–20. (London: Update Publications)
2. De Dombal, F. T. (1981). Analysis of foregut symptoms. In Baron, J. H. and Moody, F. G. (eds.) *International Medical Review: Gastroenterology I, Foregut*, pp. 49–66. (London: Butterworth)
3. Lennard Jones, J. E. (1983). Functional gastrointestinal disorders. *N. Engl. J. Med.*, **308**, 431–435
4. Doll, R., Jones, F. A. and Bukatzsch, M. M. (1950). MRC Special Report Series no. 276, London
5. Watkinson, G. (1960). The incidence of chronic peptic ulcer found at necropsy. *Gut* **1**, 14–31
6. Ihamaki, T., Varis, K. and Siurala, M. (1979). Morphological, functional and immunological state of gastric mucosa in gastric carcinoma families. Comparison with a computer matched family sample. *Scand. J. Gastroenterol.*, **14**, 801–812
7. Pulvertaft, C. N. (1968). Comments on the incidence and natural history of gastric and duodenal ulcer. *Postgrad. Med. J.*, **44**, 597–602
8. Bonnevie, O. (1975). The incidence of gastric ulcer in Copenhagen County. *Gastroenterology*, **10**, 231–239
9. Bonnevie, O. (1975). The incidence of duodenal ulcer in Copenhagen County. *Gastroenterology*, **10**, 385–393
10. Kurata, J. H., Honda, G. D. and Frankl, H. (1983). The incidence of gastric and duodenal ulcers in a large HMO. Presented at the *111th Annual Meeting of the American Public Health Association* (abstract)
11. National Centre for Health Statistics. (1979). Prevalence of selected chronic digestive conditions, United States 1975. *Vital and Health Statistics*, Department of Health, Education and Welfare, 79–1558

12. Brinton, W. (1857). *On the Pathology, Symptoms and Treatment of Ulcer of the Stomach*. (Edinburgh: Churchill Livingstone)
13. Coggon, D., Lambert, P. and Langman, M. J. S. (1981). Twenty years of hospital admissions for peptic ulcer in England and Wales. *Lancet*, **1**, 1302–1304
14. Elashoff, J. D. and Grossman, M. I. (1980). Trends in hospital admissions and death rates from peptic ulcer in the United States from 1970–1978. *Gastroenterology*, **78**, 280–285
15. Almy, T. P. *et al.* (1975). Prevalence and significance of digestive disease. *Gastroenterology*, **68**, 1351–1371
16. Mendeloff, A. I. (1974). What has been happening to duodenal ulcer? *Gastroenterology*, **64**, 1020–1022
17. Vogt, T. M. and Johnson, R. E. (1980). Recent changes in the incidence of duodenal and gastric ulcer. *Am. J. Epidemiol.*, **111**, 713–720
18. Taylor, P. (1974). Sickness absence; Facts and misconceptions. *J. R. Coll. Physicians, London*, **8**, 315–333
19. Kurata, J. H. and Haile, B. M. (1984). Epidemiology of peptic disease. *Clin. Gastroenterol.*, 13:2, 289–307
20. Malhotra, S. L. (1965). The role of saliva in the aetiology of peptic ulcer. *Br. Med. J.*, **1**, 1220–1222
21. Langman, M. J. S. (1979). *The Epidemiology of Chronic Digestive Disease*. (London: Edward Arnold)
22. Harrison, A., Elashoff, J. and Grossman, M. I. (1979). Cigarette smoking and ulcer disease. In *The Surgeon General's Report on Smoking and Health*, pp. 9–21. (US Department of Health, Education and Welfare, Public Health Service)
23. Paffenbarger, R. S., Wing, A. L. and Hyde, R. T. (1974). Chronic disease in former college students. *Am. J. Epidemiol.*, **100**, 307–315
24. Petitti, D. B., Friedman, G. D. and Kahn, W. (1982). Peptic ulcer disease and the tar and nicotine yield of currently smoked cigarettes. *J. Chronic Dis.*, **35**, 503–507
25. Hammond, E. C. (1966). Smoking in relation to the death rates of one million men and women. In Haenszel, W. (ed.) *Epidemiological Approaches to the Study of Cancer and Other Chronic Diseases*. National Cancer Institute Monograph **19**, pp. 127–204. (Bethesda: US Public Health Service)
26. Friedman, G. D., Siegelaub, A. B. and Seltzer, C. C. (1974). Cigarettes, alcohol, coffee and peptic ulcer. *N. Engl. J. Med.*, **290**, 469–473
27. Doll, R., Jones, F. and Pygott, F. (1958). Effect of smoking on the production and maintenance of gastric and duodenal ulcers. *Lancet*, **1**, 657–662
28. Gugler, R., Rohner, H. G., Kratochvil, P. *et al.* (1982). Effect of smoking on duodenal ulcer healing with cimetidine and oxmetidine. *Gut*, **23**, 866–871
29. Peterson, W. L., Sturdevant, R. A. L., Frankl, H. D. *et al.* (1977). Healing of duodenal ulcer with an antacid regimen. *N. Engl. J. Med.*, **297**, 341–345
30. Korman, M. G., Hansky, J., Eaves, E. R. and Schmidt, G. T. (1983).

Influence of cigarette smoking on healing and relapse in duodenal ulcer disease. *Gastroenterology*, **85**, 871–874

31. Read, N. W. and Grech, P. (1973). Effect of cigarette smoking on competence of the pylorus: preliminary study. *Br. Med. J.*, **3**, 313–316

32. Valenzuela, J., Defelippi, C. and Csendes, A. (1976). Manometric studies on the human pyloric sphincter. *Gastroenterology*, **70**, 481–483

33. Murthy, S., Dinoso, V., Clearfield, H. and Chey, W. (1977). Simultaneous measurement of basal pancreatic, gastric acid secretion, plasma gastrin and secretion during smoking. *Gastroenterology*, **73**, 758–761

34. McCready, D. R., Clark, L. and Cohen, M. M. (1985). Cigarette smoking reduces human gastric luminal prostaglandin E2. *Gut*, **26**, 1192–1196

35. Piper, D. W., McIntosh, J. H., Greig, M. and Shy, C. M. (1982). Environmental factors and chronic gastric ulcer: a case control study of the association of smoking, alcohol and heavy analgesic ingestion with the exacerbation of chronic gastric ulcer. *Scand. J. Gastroenterol.*, **17**, 721–729

36. Langman, M. J. S. and Cooke, A. R. (1976). Gastric and duodenal ulcer and their associated diseases. *Lancet*, **1**, 680–683

37. Cohen, S. and Booth, G. H. Jr. (1975). Gastric acid secretion and lower oesophageal sphincter pressure in response to coffee and caffeine. *N. Engl. J. Med.*, **293**, 897–899

38. Jorgensen, T. G. and Gyntelberg, F. (1976). Occurrence of peptic ulcer disease in Copenhagen males age 40–59. *Danish Medical Bulletin*, **23**, 23–28

39. Truelove, S. C. (1960). Stilboestrol, phenobarbitone and diet in chronic duodenal ulcer. *Br. Med. J.*, **2**, 559

40. Doll, R. (1964). Medical treatment of gastric ulcer. *Scott. Med. J.*, **9**(5), 183–196

41. Buchman, E., Kaung, D. T., Dolan, K. and Knapp, R. N. (1969). Unrestricted diet in the treatment of duodenal ulcer. *Gastroenterology*, **56**(6), 1016–1026

42. Malhotra, S. L. (1978). A comparison of unrefined meat and rice diets in the management of duodenal ulcer. *Postgrad. Med. J.*, **54**, 6–9

43. Rydning, A., Berstad, A., Aadland, E. and Odegaard, B. (1982). Prophylactic effect of dietary fibre in duodenal ulcer disease. *Lancet*, **2**, 736–739

44. Billington, B. P. (1963). The Australian gastric ulcer change: interstate variations. *Aust. Ann. Med.*, **12**, 153–159

45. Levy, M. (1974). Aspirin use in patients with major upper gastrointestinal bleeding and peptic ulcer disease. *N. Engl. J. Med.*, **290**, 1158–1162

46. Davenport, H. W. (1967). Salicylate damage to the gastric mucosal barrier. *N. Engl. J. Med.*, **276**, 1307

47. Vane, J. R. (1976). Inhibition of prostaglandin synthesis as a mechanism of action for aspirin-like drugs. *Nature*, **231**, 232–235

48. Conn, H. O. and Blitzer, B. I. (1976). Medical progress: non-association of adrenocorticosteroid therapy and peptic ulcer. *N. Engl. J. Med.*, **294**, 473

49. Messer, J., Reitman, D., Sacks, H. S. *et al.* (1983). Association of adreno-corticoid therapy and peptic ulcer disease. *N. Engl. J. Med.*, **309**, 21–24

50. Sommerville, K., Faulkner, G., Langman, M. (1986). Non-steroidal anti-inflammatory drugs and bleeding peptic ulcer. *Lancet*, **1**, 462–464

51. Collier, D. St J. and Pain, J. A. (1985). Non-steroidal anti-inflammatory drugs and peptic ulcer perforation. *Gut*, **26**, 359–363

52. Walt, R., Katschinski, B., Logan, R. *et al.* (1986). Rising frequency of ulcer perforation in elderly people in the United Kingdom. *Lancet*, **1**, 489–492

53. Wolf, S. and Wolff, H. G. (1943). *Human Gastric Function*, 1st Edn. (New York: Oxford University Press)

54. Peters, M. N. and Richardson, C. T. (1983). Stressful life events, acid hypersecretion and ulcer disease. *Gastroenterology*, **84**, 114–119

55. Thomas, J., Grieg, M. and Piper, D. W. (1980). Chronic gastric ulcer and life events. *Gastroenterology*, **78**, 905–911

56. Piper, D. W., McIntosh, J. H., Ariotti, D. E. *et al.* (1981). Life events and chronic duodenal ulcer: a case control study. *Gut*, **22**, 1011–1017

57. Feldman, E. J., Elashoff, J. D., Samloff, I. M. and Grossman, M. I. (1980). Psychologic stress and duodenal ulcer. *N. Engl. J. Med.*, **302**, 1206

58. Weiner, H., Thaler, M., Reiser, M. E. and Mirsky, I. A. (1957). Etiology of duodenal ulcer: relation of specific psychological characteristics to rate of gastric secretion (serum pepsinogen). *Psychosom. Med.*, **24**, 398–416

59. Rotter, J. I. Peptic ulcer. In Emery, A. E. H. and Rimoin, D. L. (eds.) *Principles and Practice of Medical Genetics*, pp. 863–878 (Edinburgh: Churchill Livingstone)

60. Langman, M. J. S. (1973). Blood group and alimentary disorders. *Clin. Gastroenterol.*, **2**, 497–506

61. Sturdevant, R. A. L., Isenberg, J. L., Secrist, D. and Ansfield, J. (1977). Antacid and placebo produced similar pain relief in duodenal ulcer patients. *Gastroenterology*, **72**, 1–5

62. Lorber, S. H., Stelzer, F. A. and Mayer, E. M. (1978). Effect of antacid and placebo on pain of duodenal ulcer. *Gastroenterology*, **74**, 1058

63. Rune, S. J. and Zachariasson, A. (1980). Acute relief of epigastric pain by antacid in duodenal ulcer patients. *Scand. J. Gastroenterol.* (supplement), **15**, 41–45

64. Peterson, W. L., Sturdevant, R. A. L., Frankl, H. D. *et al.* (1977). Healing of duodenal ulcer with an antacid regimen. *N. Engl. J. Med.*, **297**, 341–345

65. Lam, S. K., Lam, K. C., Lai, C. L. *et al.* (1979). Treatment of duodenal ulcer with antacid and sulpiride: A double blind study. *Gastroenterology*, 315–322

66. Berstad, A., Rydning, A., Aadland, E. *et al.* (1982). Controlled clinical

trial of duodenal ulcer healing with antacid tablets. *Scand. J. Gastroenterol.*, **17**(7): 953–959

67. Cayer, D., Sohmer, M. F. and Ruffin, J. M. (1957). The effect of prolonged continuous therapy on the course of chronic recurrent peptic ulcer: antacid therapy with dihydroxy aluminium aminoacetate (alglyn). *N. Carolina Med. J.*, **18**, 315–317

68. Baker, L. R. I., Ackrill, P., Catell, W. R. *et al.* (1974). Iatrogenic osteomalacia and myopathy due to phosphate depletion. *Br. Med. J.*, **iii**, 150–152

69. Spencer, H. and Lender, M. (1979). Adverse effects of aluminium-containing antacids on mineral metabolism. *Gastroenterology*, **76**, 603–606

70. Fordtran, J. S. (1968). Acid rebound. *N. Engl. J. Med.*, **279**, 900–905

71. Barry, R. E. and Ford, J. (1978). Sodium content and neutralizing capacity of some commonly used antacids. *Br. Med. J.*, **276**, 413

72. Ekenved, G., Magnusson, A., Bodemar, G. and Walan, A. (1977). Influence of food on the effect of propantheline and 1-hyoscyamine on salivation. *Scand. J. Gastroenterol.*, **12**, 963–966

73. Post, C. and Walan, A. Influence of food on the effect of 1-hyoscyamine and benzilonium-bromide in man. *Scand. J. Gastroenterol.* **45**, (Suppl.) 77

74. Ivey, K. J. (1978). Anticholinergics: do they work in peptic ulcer? *Gastroenterology*, **68**, 154–166

75. Feldman, M., Richardson, C. T., Peterson, W. L. *et al.* (1977). Effect of low dose propantheline on food stimulated acid secretion. *N. Engl. J. Med.*, **297**, 1427–1430

76. Hammer, R., Berrie, C. P., Birdsall, N. J. M. *et al.* (1980). Pirenzipine distinguishes between different subclasses of muscarinic receptors. *Nature*, **283**, 90–92

77. Stenquist, B., Hagland, U., Lind, T. and Olbe, L. (1982). The effect of different anticholinergics on the gastric acid response to sham feeding in man. *Scand. J. Gastroenterol.* **72**, (Suppl.), 165–167

78. Texter, E. C. and Reilly, P. A. (1982). The efficacy and selectivity of pirenzipine. Review and commentary. Scand. J. Gastroenterol., **72**, (Suppl.), 237–246

79. Adami, H. O., Bjorklund, O., Enander, L. K. *et al.* (1982). Cimetidine or propantheline combined with antacid therapy for short term treatment of duodenal ulcer. *Dig. Dis. Sci.*, **27**(5), 388–393

80. Ström, M., Gotthard, R., Bodemar, G. and Walan, A. (1981). Antacid/anti-cholinergic, cimetidine and placebo in treatment of active peptic ulcers. *Scand. J. Gastroenterol.*, **16**, 593–602

81. Meeroff, M., Serchio, A. and Tagablue, N. R. (1981). Anticholinergic and antacid tablets versus cimetidine in the treatment of active duodenal ulcers. *Curr. Ther. Res.*, **29**(6), 866–873

82. Walan, A. (1984). Antacids and anticholinergics in the treatment of duodenal ulcer. In Isenberg, J. I. and Johansson, C. (eds.) *Peptic Ulcer Disease*, Clinics in Gastroenterology, pp. 473–499 (London: Saunders)

83. Dal Monte, P. R., Bianchi Porro, G., Petrulo, M. *et al.* (1982). Long term treatment of duodenal ulcer with pirenzipine. A double blind placebo controlled trial. *Scand. J. Gastroenterol.,* **72,** (Suppl.), 225–227

84. Pounder, R. E., Williams, J. G., Russell, R. C. G. *et al.* (1976). Inhibition of food-stimulated gastric acid secretion by cimetidine. *Gut,* **17,** 161–168

85. Walt, R. P., Male, P-J, Rawlings, J. *et al.* (1981). Comparison of the effects of ranitidine, cimetidine and placebo on the 24 hour intragastric acidity and nocturnal acid secretion in patients with duodenal ulcer. *Gut,* **22,** 49–54

86. Thomas, J. M. and Misiewicz, G. (1984) Histamine H_2 receptor antagonists in the short and long-term treatment of duodenal ulcer. In Isenberg, J. I. and Johansson, C. (eds.) *Peptic Ulcer Disease,* Clinics in Gastroenterology, pp. 501–541 (London: W. B. Saunders).

87. Malchow, H., Sewing, K. F., Albinus, M. *et al.* (1978). In-patient treatment of peptic ulcer with cimetidine 1. Effect on the healing of duodenal ulcer. *Deutsche Medizinische Wochenschrift,* **103,** 149–152

88. Villalobos, J. J., Elizondo, J., Guevara, L. and Centeno, F. (1978). Cimetidine in the treatment of duodenal ulcer: Double blind study. *J. Int. Med. Res.,* **6,** 351

89. Pounder, R. E. (1981). Model of medical treatment for duodenal ulcer. *Lancet,* **1:** 29–30

90. Capurso, L., Dal Monte, P. R., Mazzeo, F. *et al.* (1984). Comparison of cimetidine 800 mg once daily and 400 mg twice daily in acute duodenal ulceration. *Br. Med. J.,* **289,** 1418–1420

91. Isenberg, J. I., Peterson, W. L., Elashoff, J. D. *et al.* (1983). Healing of benign gastric ulcer with low dose antacid or cimetidine. A double blind randomized placebo-controlled trial. *N. Engl. J. Med.,* **308,** 1319–1324

92. Akdamar, K., Dyke, W., Englert, E. *et al.* (1981). Cimetidine versus placebo in the treatment of benign gastric ulcer: a multi-centre double blind study. *Gastroenterology,* **80,** 1098 (abstract)

93. Ashton, M. G., Holdsworth, C. D., Ryan, F. P. and Moore, M. (1982). Healing of gastric ulcers after one, two and three months of ranitidine. *Br. Med. J.,* **284,** 467–468

94. Wright, J. P., Marks, I. N., Mee, A. S. *et al.* (1982). Ranitidine in the treatment of gastric ulceration. *S. Afr. J. Med.,* **61,** 155–158

95. Ireland, A., Colin Jones, D. G., Gear, P. *et al.* (1984). Ranitidine 150 mg twice daily vs 300 mg nightly in treatment of duodenal ulcers. *Lancet,* **2,** 274–276

96. Lishman, A. H. and Record, C. O. (1982) Ranitidine in the management of duodenal ulceration: controlled and open comparison with cimetidine. In Misiewicz, J. J. and Wormsley, K. G. (eds.) *The Clinical Use of Ranitidine.* Proceedings of the Second International Symposium on Ranitidine 1982, pp. 163–167. (Oxford: Medicine Publishing Foundation)

97. Witzel, L. and Wolberg, E. (1982). Peptic ulcer healing with ranitidine in cimetidine resistance. *Lancet*, **2:** 1224
98. Bardhan, K. D. (1980). Cimetidine in duodenal ulcer: the present position. In Torsoli, A., Luchelli, P. E. and Brimblecombe, R. W. (eds.) *Further Experience with H₂ Receptor Antagonists in Peptic Ulcer Disease and Progress in Histamine Research*, pp. 5–14 (Amsterdam: Excerpta Medica)
99. Hunt, R. H. (1981). Non responders to cimetidine treatment part 1. In Baron, J. H. (ed.) *Cimetidine in the 80's*, pp. 34–41. (Edinburgh: Churchill Livingstone)
100. Gough, K. R., Korman, M. G., Bardhan, K. D. *et al*. (1984). Ranitidine and cimetidine in prevention of duodenal ulcer relapse. A double blind randomized multicentre comparative trial. *Lancet*, **2**, 659–662
101. Roth, H. P. (1971). Healing of initial ulcers in relation of age and sex. *Gastroenterology*, **61**, 570–575
102. Jensen, K. B., Milmann, K. M., Rahbek, I. *et al*. (1979). Prophylactic effect of cimetidine in gastric ulcer patients. *Scand. J. Gastroenterol.*, **14**, 175–176
103. Machell, R. J., Ciclitira, P. J., Farthing, M. J. *et al*. (1979). Cimetidine in the prevention of gastric ulcer relapse. *Postgrad. Med.*, **55**, 393–395
104. Cockel, R., Dawson, J. and Jain, S. (1982). Ranitidine in the long term treatment of gastric ulcers. In Misiewicz, J. J. and Wormsley, K. G. (eds.), *The Clinical Use of Cimetidine*, pp. 232–238. (Oxford: Medicine Publishing Foundation)
105. Zamcheek, N., Grable, E., Ley, A. and Norman, L. (1955). Occurrence of gastric cancer among patients with pernicious anaemia at Boston City Hospital. *N. Engl. J. Med.*, **252**, 1103–1110
106. Domellöf, L., Eriksson, S. and Janunger, K. G. (1977). Carcinoma and possible pre-cancerous changes of the gastric stump after Billroth II resection. *Gastroenterology*, **73**, 462–468
107. Tannenbaum, S. R. (1983). N-nitroso compounds: a perspective on human exposure. *Lancet*, **1**, 629–632
108. Habs, M., Schmähl, D., Eisenbrand, G. and Preussmann, R. (1983). Carcinogenesis studies with N-nitrosocimetidine. In Magee, P. N. (ed.) *Nitrosamines and Human Cancer*, Banbury Report No. 12, pp. 403–405. (New York: Cold Spring Harbor Laboratory)
109. Lijinsky, W. (1982). Carcinogenesis studies with nitrosocimetidine. In Magee, P. N. (ed.) *Nitrosamines and Human Cancer*. Banbury Report No. 12, pp. 397–401, (New York: Cold Spring Harbor Laboratory)
110. Colin Jones, D. G., Langman, M. J. S., Dawson, D. H. and Vessey, M. P. (1985). Postmarketing surveillance of the safety of cimetidine mortality during second, third and fourth years of follow-up. *Br. Med. J.*, **291**, 1084–1088
111. Buck, J. P., Murgatroyd, R. E., Bolston, A. W. and Baron, J. H. (1979). Perforation of gastric carcinoma (at site of previous benign ulcer) after withdrawal of cimetidine. *Lancet*, **2**, 42
112. Reed, P. I., Cassell, P. G. and Walters, C. L. (1979). Gastric cancer in patients who have taken cimetidine. *Lancet*, **1**, 1234–1235

113. Taylor, T. V., Lee, D., Howatson, A. G. *et al.* (1979). Gastric cancer and cimetidine. *J. R. Coll. Surg. Edinburgh*, **26**, 34–35

114. Walan, A., Bergasker-Aspoy, J., Farup, P., *et al.* (1983). Four week study of the rate of duodenal ulcer healing with omeprazole. *Gut*, **24**, A972

115. Lauritson, K., Rune, S. J., Bytzer, P. *et al.* (1985). Effect of omeprazole and cimetidine on duodenal ulcer. A double blind comparative trial. *N. Engl. J. Med.*, **312**, 958–961

116. Nagashima, R. (1981). Mechanisms of action of sucralfate. *J. Clin. Gastroenterol.*, **3** (Suppl. 2), 117–127

117. Sasaki, H., Hinohara, Y., Tsunoda, Y. and Nagashima, R. (1983). Binding of sucralfate to duodenal ulcer in man. *Scand. J. Gastroenterol.*, **18** (Suppl. 83) 13–14

118. McGraw, B. F. and Caldwell, E. G. (1981). Sucralfate. *Drug Intell. Clin. Pharm.*, **15**, 578–580

119. Garnett, W. R. (1982). Sucralfate – alternative therapy for peptic ulcer disease. *Clin. Pharm.*, *1*, 307-314

120. Samloff, I. M., O'Dell, C. (1985). Inhibition of peptic activity by sucralfate. *Am. J. Med.*, **79**: (Suppl. 2c) 15–18

121. Fixa, B. and Komárková, O. (1981). Aluminium sucrose sulphate (sucralfate) in the treatment of peptic ulcer (double blind study). In Caspary, W. F. (ed.) *Sucralfate: A New Therapeutic Concept*, pp. 80–84, (Baltimore: Urban and Schwarzenberg)

122. McHardy, G. G. (1981). A multicentre double blind trial of sucralfate and placebo in duodenal ulcer. *J. Clin. Gastroenterol.*, **3**, (Suppl. 2) 147–152

123. Tytgat, G. N. J., Hameeteman, W., Van Olffen, G. H. (1984). Miscellaneous Drugs. In Isenberg, J. I. and Johansson, C. (eds.), *Peptic Ulcer Disease*, Clinics in Gastroenterology, pp. 543–568, (London: W. B. Saunders)

124. Brandstaetter, G. and Kratochvil, P. (1985). Comparison of sucralfate dosages (2 g twice a day versus 1 g four times a day) in duodenal ulcer healing. *Am. J. Med.*, **79**: (Suppl. 2c) 36–38

125. Marks, I. N., Wright, J. P., Denyer, M. *et al.* (1980). Comparison of sucralfate with cimetidine in the short-term treatment of chronic peptic ulcer. *S. Afr. Med. J.* **57**, 567–573

126. Lahtinen, J., Ankee, S., Miettinen, P. *et al.* (1983). Sucralfate and cimetidine for gastric ulcer. *Scand. J. Gastroenterol.*, **18**, (Suppl. 83) 49–51

127. Classen, M., Bethge, H., Brunner, G. *et al.* (1982). Sucralfate prevents duodenal ulcer recurrences. A controlled double blind study. *Gastroenterology*, **82**, 1034

128. Libeskind, M. (1982). Maintenance treatment of patients with healed peptic ulcer with sucralfate, placebo and cimetidine. *Scand. J. Gastroenterol.*, **18**, (Suppl. 83) 69–70

129. Marks, I. N., Wright, J. P., Girdwood, A. H. *et al.* (1985). Maintenance therapy with sucralfate reduces rate of gastric ulcer recurrence. *Am. J. Med.*, **79** (Suppl. 2c) 32–35

130. Lee, S. P. (1982). A potential mechanism of action of colloidal bismuth subcitrate: diffusion barrier to hydrochloric acid. *Scand. J. Gastroenterol.*, **17**, (Suppl. 80) 17–21

131. Brogden, R. N., Pinder, R. M., Sawyer, P. R. *et al.* (1976). Tripotassium dicitratobismuthate: a report of its pharmacological properties and therapeutic efficacy in peptic ulcer. *Drugs,* **12**, 401–411

132. Boyes, B. E., Woolf, I. L., Wilson, R. Y. *et al.* (1975). Treatment of gastric ulceration with a bismuth preparation. *Postgrad. Med. J.,* **51** (Suppl. 5) 29–32

133. Lee, S. P. and Nicholson, G. I. (1977). Increased healing of gastric and duodenal ulcer in a controlled trial using tripotassium dicitratobismuthate. *Med. J. Aust.,* **1**, 808–812

134. Tytgat, G. N. J., Van Bentem, N. Van Olffen, G. *et al.* (1982). Controlled trial comparing colloidal bismuth subcitrate tablets, cimetidine and placebo in the treatment of gastric ulceration. *Scand. J. Gastroenterol.,* **17**, (Suppl. 80) 31–38

135. Martin, D. F., Hollanders, D., May, S. J. *et al.* (1981). Difference in relapse rates of duodenal ulcer after healing with cimetidine or tripotassium dicitratobismuthate. *Lancet,* **1**, 7–10

136. Lee, F. I., Samloff, T. M. and Hardman, M. (1985). Comparison of tripotassium dicitratobismuthate tablets with ranitidine in healing and relapse of duodenal ulcers. *Lancet,* **1**, 1229–1230

137. Kang, J. Y. and Piper, D. N., (1982). Cimetidine and colloidal bismuth in the treatment of chronic duodenal ulcer: comparison of initial healing and recurrence after healing. *Digestion,* **23**, 73–79

138. Archambault, A. P., Halvorsen, L., Lee, S. P. *et al.* (1984). Efficacy and safety of enprostil, a synthetic prostaglandin and placebo in patients with duodenal ulcer. *Am. J. Gastroenterol.,* **79**, 828

139. Lauritsen, K., Laursen, L. S., Havelund, T. *et al.* (1986). Effect of enprostil and ranitidine on duodenal ulcer healing. *Gut,* **27**, A608

140. Walt, R. P., Long, R. G., Logan, R. F. A. *et al.* (1986). Double blind clinical trial comparing night time enprostil with ranitidine in duodenal ulcer. *Gut,* **27**, A608

141. Sontag, S., Graham, D. Y., Belsito, A. *et al.* (1984). Cimetidine, cigarette smoking and recurrence of duodenal ulcer. *N. Engl. J. Med.,* **311**, 689–693

142. Cumberland, D. C. (1975). Fibreoptic endoscopy and radiology in the investigation of the upper gastrointestinal tract. *Clin. Radiol.,* **26**, 223–236

143. Barnes, R. J., Gear, M. W. L., Nicol, A. and Drew, A. B. (1974). Study of dyspepsia in a general practice as assessed by endoscopy and radiology. *Br. Med. J.,* **4**, 214–216

144. Laufer, I., Mullens, J. E. and Hamilton, J. (1975). The diagnostic accuracy of barium studies of the stomach and duodenum – correlation with endoscopy. *Radiology,* **115**, 569–573

145. Shirakabe, H., Nishizawa, M., Nomoto, K. *et al.* (1975). Qualitative comparison of endoscopy and radiology in the diagnosis of duodenal ulcer. *Gastroenterology,* **68**, 1031

146. Fraser, G. M. and Earnshaw, P. M. (1983). The double contrast barium meal: a correlation with endoscopy. *Clin. Radiol.*, **34**, 121-131
147. Cotton, P. B. and Shorvon, P. J. (1984). Endoscopy and radiology in peptic ulcer disease. In Isenberg, J. I. and Johansson, C. (eds.), *Peptic Ulcer Disease*, Clinics in Gastroenterology, pp. 383–403, (London: W. B. Saunders)
148. Farini, R., Farinati, F., Cardin, F. *et al.* (1983). Evidence of gastric carcinoma during follow-up of apparently benign gastric ulcer. *Gut*, **24**, A486
149. Schiller, K. F. R. and Prout, B. J. (1976). Hazards. In Schiller, K. F. R. and Salmon, P. R. (eds.) *Modern Topics in Gastrointestinal Endoscopy*, pp. 147–165, (London: William Heinemann Medical)
150. Holdstock, C. D., Bardhan, K. D. and Balmforth, G. V. (1979). Upper gastrointestinal endoscopy: its effect on patient management. *Br. Med. J.*, **1**, 775–777
151. Lance, P. and Gazzard, B. G. (1983). Controlled trial of cimetidine for symptomatic treatment of duodenal ulcers. *Br. Med. J.*, **286**, 937–938
152. Bardhan, K. D. (1980). Intermittent treatment of duodenal ulcer with cimetidine. *Br. Med. J.*, **2**, 20–22
153. Rune, S. J., Mollman, K. M. and Rahbek, J. (1980). Frequency of relapses in duodenal ulcer patients treated with cimetidine during symptomatic periods. *Scand. J. Gastroenterol.*, **15** (Suppl. 58) 85–92
154. Fry, J. (1964). Peptic ulcer: a profile. *Br. Med. J.*, **2**, 809–812
155. Kraus, E. (1963). Long term results of medical and surgical treatment. A follow-up investigation of patients initially treated conservatively between 1925 and 1934. *Acta. Chir. Scand.* (Suppl. 310).
156. Viskum, K. (1976). A comparison of the course of the disease among patients with gastric ulcer, duodenal ulcer and ulcer dyspepsia without ulcer demonstrable by X-ray. *Dan. Med. Bull.*, **23**, 129–136
157. Mazzaca, G., D'Agostino, L., D'Arienzo, A. *et al.* (1982). Cimetidine or ranitidine non-responder patients. Treatment of duodenal ulcers resistant to one H_2 blocker with the other. *Scand. J. Gastroenterol.*, **17** (Suppl. 78), 103 (abstract 408)
158. Lam, S. K., Lee, N. W., Koo, J. *et al.* (1984). Randomized crossover trial of tripotassium dicitratobismuthate versus high dose cimetidine for duodenal ulcers resistant to standard dose of cimetidine. *Gut*, **25**, 703
159. Bardhan, K. D., Thompson, M., Bose, K. *et al.* (1986). Combined histamine H_2 and antimuscarinic receptor blockade in the treatment of refractory duodenal ulcer. *Gut*, **27**, A606
160. Gustavsson, S., Adami, H. O., Lööf, A. *et al.* (1983). Rapid healing of duodenal ulcers with omeprazole: a double blind dose-comparative trial. *Lancet*, **2**, 124–125
161. Gear, M. W. L. (1986). The place of surgery in the management of peptic ulcer. A comparison with modern drug therapy. In Lancaster Smith, M. J. (ed.) *Peptic Ulcer*, Seminar, pp. 13–22 (London: Update Siebart Publications)
162. Fineberg, H. V. and Pearlman, L. A. (1981). Surgical treatment of

peptic ulcer in the United States. Trends after the introduction of cimetidine. *Lancet*, **1**, 1305–1308
163. Wastell, C. (1982). The stomach and duodenum. In Bouchier, I.A.D. (ed.) *Recent Advances in Gastroenterology*, **33** (Edinburgh: Churchill Livingstone)
164. Johnston, D. (1975). Operative mortality and morbidity of highly selective vagotomy, **4**, 545–547
165. Clark, C. G. (1982). Recurrent ulcer. In Barron, J. H., Alexander-Williams, J., Allgower, M., Muller, C. and Spencer, J. (eds.) *Vagotomy in Modern Surgical Practice*, pp. 305–332 (London: Butterworths)
166. Kennedy, T. L. (1982). Recurrent ulcer. In Barron, J. H., Alexander-Williams, J., Allgower, M., Muller, C. and Spencer, J. (eds.) *Vagotomy in Modern Surgical Practice*, pp. 327–329 (London: Butterworths)
167. Kelly, K. A. and Malagelada, J. R. (1984). Medical and surgical treatment of chronic gastric ulcer. In Isenberg, J. I. and Johansson, C. (eds.) *Peptic Ulcer*, Clinics in Gastroenterology, pp. 621–634 (London: W. B. Saunders)
168. Duthie, H. L. and Kwong, N. K. (1973). Vagotomy or gastrectomy for gastric ulcer. *Br. Med. J.*, **4**, 79–81
169. Poppen, B. and Delin, A. (1981). Parietal cell vagotomy for duodenal and pyloric ulcers. I. Clinical factors leading to failure of the operation. *Am. J. Surg.*, **141**, 323–329
170. Barron, J. H., Barr, J., Batten, J., Sidebottom, R. and Spencer, J. (1986). Acid, pepsin and mucus secretion in patients with gastric and duodenal ulcer before and after colloidal bismuth Subcitrate (Denol). *Gut*, **27**, 486–490

4

NON-ULCER DYSPEPSIA

J. G. C. KINGHAM

INTRODUCTION

Dyspepsia is a term which covers a multitude of symptoms and has no commonly agreed definition. It is often used inter-changeably with indigestion, but has a pseudo scientific ring to it which may be useful in reassuring the patient that his condition is taken seriously, but may unfortunately delude the doctor into believing he has a greater understanding of the patient's condition than is actually the case. A survey[1] con-ducted recently amongst groups of senior hospital doctors and patients with a variety of gastroenterological and non-gastroenterological disorders showed that there was much confusion as to what dyspepsia and indigestion implied. It seems that doctors by and large consider both terms to describe those symptoms typically associated with peptic ulceration. Most patients, on the other hand, though sometimes using the term dyspepsia, are uncertain what it means and are more conversant with indigestion. Unlike their medical counter-parts, they are not familiar with the classical symptoms of peptic ulcer and give a less fettered account of what indigestion entails. Many of the symptoms which patients in that survey listed as indigestion, whether they were perennial or only occasional sufferers, more closely resembled irritable bowel syndrome than peptic ulceration. In this study[1] we were careful not to bias our findings in favour of the hypothesis that indigestion may equate with a functional bowel disorder by excluding patients with such a diagnosis. The study revealed that 80% of those questioned suffered occasional indigestion. Only half of the patients understood what dyspepsia meant, but most of the doctors considered that indigestion and dyspepsia were synonymous. Not surprisingly, around four-fifths of the patients and doctors included upper abdominal pain, wind, heartburn and acid regurgitation as typical indigestion/dyspepsia symptoms. More surprisingly, over half of the patients listed lower abdominal pain and irregular bowel habit, especially constipation, as characteristic features of indigestion and just less than half also included headache and backache. The majority considered that predominant causes were heavy meals, over spiced food, alcohol and worry. A similar proportion felt that relief was best achieved by taking antacids or laxatives, particularly if the preparation induced belching. Interestingly the patients, unlike the doctors, did not accept that drinking milk was likely to give relief.

Having accepted that dyspepsia defies precise definition, it can still be said, from the example of the study cited above[1] and the accumulated clinical experience of a host of others, that the condition encompasses some or all of the following symptoms: (1) abdominal pain, (2) abdominal fullness or discomfort, (3) wind, (4) heartburn and (5) nausea. Other rather poorly defined symptoms are often mentioned such as leaden sensation or lump in the stomach, acidity and an unpleasant taste in the mouth. In addition, some consider vomiting and bowel dysfunction to be an integral part of dyspepsia. Such a broad spectrum of interpretation of course devalues the term and in a medical sense it can only be viewed as implying a disturbance of the digestive tract with greater emphasis on its upper than its lower reaches. A working definition of dyspepsia has been proposed by workers from the Southern General Hospital in Glasgow[2] who have made analysis of dyspepsia their raison d'être: episodic, recurrent or persistent abdominal pain or discomfort or any other symptom referable to the alimentary tract except rectal bleeding or jaundice.

It should now be apparent that non-ulcer dyspepsia does not assume typical ulcer symptoms in the absence of ulceration. In medical parlance, the description is used in two separate circumstances. Firstly, it may be the clinical impression after interviewing the patient either before, or often without, investigation. The implication here is that the dyspeptic symptoms did not clinically suggest a peptic ulcer nor any other serious pathology. In these circumstances, the description does not necessarily exclude an organic diagnosis, though experience shows that an organic basis for the symptoms is less likely to be unearthed. An analysis of the actual symptoms, a full medical and drug history and knowledge of the age of the patient, his smoking and drinking habits and so forth will determine whether an initial impression of non-ulcer dyspepsia is appropriate. The second circumstance in which the description may be used is to categorize patients with diverse symptoms which may or may not have suggested peptic ulceration, gall stones etc., but whose subsequent investigations have failed to reveal any abnormality. I believe it is confusing to include within the concept of non-ulcer dyspepsia conditions with a well-defined organic basis which can present with upper gastrointestinal symptoms. I, therefore, intend to exclude from further discussion peptic oesophagitis, achalasia of the cardia, inflammatory bowel disease, pancreatitis, cholangitis and angina. On the other hand, I propose to further analyse the following: (1) conditions with an uncertain organic basis such as motility disorders of the upper G.I. tract and biliary dyskinesia, (2) conditions with a well-defined pathological basis, but ill-defined or absent clinical correlates such as chronic cholecystitis, gastritis and duodenitis and (3) conditions which are often misinterpreted or misconceived such as cholelithiasis and hiatus hernia.

The Extent of the Problem

What is the distribution of disease in patients presenting with dyspepsia as defined by the Glasgow school? The results, of course, will always depend on local circumstances, methods of referral, diagnostic facilities and clinical acumen, but the figures from Glasgow[2] are of interest and probably fairly representative for the United Kingdom. Of 1200 referrals to their department of gastroenterology, approximately one-third had peptic ulcers, one-quarter had no organic cause found, one-sixth had typical irritable bowel syndrome and the remaining quarter had organic colonic, gastric or biliary diseases in roughly equal proportions. It should be noted that one in three patients had more than one gastrointestinal diagnosis. So in that series almost one half of the patients referred had what is loosely called a functional abnormality of the gastrointestinal tract to account for the dyspepsia. It seems a reasonable assumption that patients who are referred to hospital have worse, more persistent or more organic sounding dyspeptic symptoms than those who are not so referred. Thus the proportion of dyspeptic patients with organic disease in general practice is probably well below figures quoted for hospital surveys[3,4]. I think, at this stage, it is proper to point out that though the terms functional and non-organic are often used interchangeably, they may not be synonymous and also that conditions in which no patho-physiological disturbance can at present be demonstrated may be proven clearly organic in the light of future medical knowledge.

SYMPTOMS

The essence of diagnosis in gastroenterology lies in accurate history taking and this applies more keenly to dyspepsia than any other digestive disorder. It cannot be stressed too strongly that an extra 5 or 10 minutes extracting a detailed description of what a patient actually means by indigestion, upset tummy or acidity may save endless fruitless expeditions to X-ray departments, outpatient clinics and chemists' shops. It is a great misfortune that the ready access to sophisticated radiology and endoscopy has discouraged rather than encouraged many doctors from taking a practical clinical approach to diagnosis. Moynihan[5], in a *Lancet* article of 1905, stated that ulcer and non-ulcer dyspepsia could be easily distinguished solely on the basis of symptoms. With the advent of endoscopy, such claims have to be taken in perspective, but still the shrewd and experienced gastroenterologist should make the correct diagnosis in at least three-quarters of cases. This has been the experience of Crean and his colleagues[7] in the Glasgow dyspepsia study. Over the past dozen years, workers from Leeds[6] and Glasgow[7] using computer analysis have shown that the correct diagnosis by symptoms alone can be made in 80% of dyspeptic patients. Horrocks and De Dombal[8] have shown that this diagnostic accuracy can actually be achieved just as well by a non-medical assistant as by a skilled physician provided the appropriate questions are asked and the data properly analysed. The aim of the practitioner with a particular penchant for dyspepsia should be to make the right diagnosis on clinical grounds with the same readiness as the clerk with his computer. Many younger patients with dyspepsia can be satisfactorily diagnosed on clinical grounds alone and neither require nor benefit from investigations. All too often, in fact, investigations have a counter-productive effect, particularly in those more nervous sufferers of non-organic dyspepsia. Typically the investigations will be negative and contrary to expectation, this may not reassure the patient. He may misconstrue the negative findings in the following ways:

(1) The doctor must now believe that I am imagining my symptoms

(2) The doctor has obviously ordered the wrong investigation and is, therefore, incompetent, or

(3) I have a mysterious illness which the doctors cannot get to grips with.

In reality, (3) is almost never true, but sadly (1) and (2) frequently are. Worse still, an inappropriate investigation may provide irrelevant information leading to the wrong diagnosis[9-11]. This is likely to happen in the case of minor abnormalities which are common in the general population, but only infrequently produce symptoms. Under this heading, the top contenders are gall stones, hiatus hernia and colonic diverticulosis. It does not help a patient in any way to subject her to cholecystectomy because gall stones were found during unnecessary investigations of a typical functional dyspepsia. I will discuss symptoms individually and indicate which aspects or associations favour an organic interpretation.

PAIN

When asking the patient about his pain, it is necessary to discover the following points: (1) site, (2) radiation, (3) character, (4) intensity, (5) duration, (6) timing, (7) frequency, (8) relationship to eating and type of food, (9) relationship to eructation and passing flatus, (10) relationship to bowel movements and (11) relationship to vomiting.

Site and Radiation

Peptic ulcer pain is almost always sharply localized to the epigastrium, but may radiate to the back and either the right or the left hypochondrium. The patient will usually point to the pain accurately with one finger rather than moving the flat of his hand over a wide area of the upper abdomen. The pain of biliary colic, like peptic ulcer pain, is usually in the epigastrium though it is almost as commonly felt in the right hypochondrium. Radiation to the back and shoulder blade are fairly constant features. The pain of functional dyspepsia is predominantly in the upper abdomen, but tends to be rather

Table 4.1   Peptic ulcer pain

Epigastric – points with one finger
Episodic – prolonged remissions
At night
Relieved by food/antacids
Relieved by vomiting

poorly localized; the patient may have difficulty in demonstrating the precise position saying 'it hurts all over'. There is often pain in several abdominal areas including the lower abdomen. Such pains may be coincident or occur separately. Radiation to many extra-abdominal sites may be experienced including the back, shoulder blade and retrosternally[9,11–13]. The description of radiation to these sites should not automatically be interpreted as an indication of biliary pain, particularly if there are other features to suggest a functional gut disorder. The cardinal features of pain from peptic ulceration, biliary colic and non-ulcer dyspepsia are given in Tables 4.1–4.3.

Table 4.2   Biliary colic pain

Epigastric or right hypochondrial
Attacks few in number
Very severe with sweating/vomiting
Short duration – less than 2 hours
Crescendo–decrescendo type – not colic

Table 4.3   Functional dyspeptic pain

Poorly localized, More than one site
Constant awareness
Described severity disproportionate to clinical wellbeing
Present on waking
No relieving factors
Blamed on specific foods – especially fatty

Character and Intensity

Most of us have only a limited ability to describe a pain's quality, but the majority of patients can judge whether a pain is constant or colicky, dull, sharp or burning, mild or severe. Not infrequently patients will fail to distinguish between pain and a feeling of discomfort, uneasiness or an upset stomach. Such feelings are very common in functional dyspepsia and do not readily suggest a peptic ulcer or biliary tract disease. Peptic ulcer pain tends to be constant, though not of long duration, burning or aching and of variable severity. Colicky pain most typically arises from the intestine, but may also come from the uterus or ureter. It is unusual (less than 10%) for biliary pain to be colicky despite popular belief and the well-entrenched literal acceptance of the term biliary colic. Patients may not really understand what colicky pain implies: if they are parous women, then they should be asked if the pain comes in waves like in labour. The other useful reference point is the griping pains of food poisoning or gastroenteritis which most people have experienced at some time or another. If the pain is colicky, then it is a safe bet that the small or large gut is responsible for the symptoms and a functional aetiology is commoner than inflammation or obstruction. The severity of the pain does not discriminate well between peptic ulcer and non-ulcer dyspepsia, but if the patient is given to hyperbole in describing the symptoms, then this is a little suggestive of non-organic disease. Women who describe permanently unbearable pain making them cry out whilst in company, but who look otherwise well are unlikely to harbour a peptic ulcer. On the other hand, biliary colic is usually excruciatingly painful, enough to make the sufferer sweat and vomit, but its other characteristics (shortlived and infrequent) generally serve to differentiate it from both peptic ulcer and non-ulcer dyspepsia.

Duration, Timing and Frequency

These are important features which may help to differentiate between organic and non-organic dyspepsia. Duodenal ulcer pain typically lasts half an hour to 2 hours at a time occurring daily for a few weeks and then remitting for weeks or months at a time. Pain that comes on in the night and wakes the patient driving him to get relief from milk, a snack or antacids, is very likely to be caused by a duodenal ulcer. Pain which is present all day long from waking in the morning until going to bed at night, day in day out, in the presence of otherwise good health is much more likely to be functional than organic. Shortlived episodes of severe pain occurring infrequently with long periods of pain-free existence inbetween are unlikely to be functional and may be biliary or ureteric colic. If the pain sounds typically biliary, but persists for several hours, then pancreatitis should be considered as biliary colic rarely lasts more than 2 hours.

Relationship to Eating and Type of Food

Abdominal pain is likely to be related to food whether the organ responsible is in the upper or lower alimentary tract because eating and the attendant gastric filling is the principal physiological stimulus to all digestive activity. If the doctor bears this in mind, then he will be less likely to jump to the false conclusion that pain which comes on after food must indicate a gastroduodenal or biliary tract disorder. This does not deny that post-cibal pain is a common feature of many organic and functional upper alimentary tract disorders, but emphasizes that the pain of irritable bowel and inflammatory bowel disease may also be food related. It is assumed that the pain from the lower gastrointestinal tract is induced by reflex changes in motility rather than from food entering the lumen. Epigastric pain relieved by food is a helpful indication of duodenal ulcer, though many ulcer sufferers do not experience this phenomenon. Retrosternal discomfort or burning usually represents an oesophageal disorder, but it does not necessarily imply peptic oesophagitis. The feeling of a ball of wind retrosternally or in the epigastrium after eating is a common feature of functional dyspepsia. If heartburn is specifically associated with drinking hot, acidic, fizzy or alcoholic drinks or swallowing spicy foods such as chilli or curry, then peptic oesophagitis is very likely. If, on the other hand, the heartburn is induced equally by an irritant or a bland diet, then a functional cause is more probable. Many abdominal symptoms are induced by rich or fatty foods and certain well-known indigestible items such as onions, cucumbers, green peppers and radishes[1]. *Fatty food intolerance is experienced by about 30% of the general population and it is one of the greater failings of medical education that so many doctors who should know better both believe, and worse still, teach that fat intolerance is a particular feature of cholelithiasis.* There have been so many well-conducted studies[14-17] over the past few decades showing this to be quite untrue, that it is incomprehensible why this piece of ill-informed folklore should still be so well-entrenched. The situation is all the more difficult because, over the years, it has become 'a well-known fact' in the eyes of the lay public that fat intolerance equates with gall stones. There is no doubt from the published surveys that fat intolerance is equally prevalent amongst those with or those without gall stones. A study from Pennsylvania published in 1957[14] of 1000 consecutive patients undergoing cholecystography, a third of whom turned out to have gall stones, showed that just over 50% of both the normal and the abnormal groups had food intolerance and that 35% of each group had fatty food intolerance. A survey of hospitalized patients in Boston[15] published in 1964 showed that fat intolerance was equally distributed amongst patients with gall stones, peptic ulcer, organic bowel disease and those with functional gut disorders. In each category, about 40% of patients admitted to fat intolerance. More recently, and nearer to home, two large studies, one from Wales[16] and one from Edinburgh[17], have amply confirmed the high prevalence of fat intolerance and its non-association with gall bladder disease. In my own experience, though I do not have published evidence to support this, fat intolerance is rather more common in those with functional than those with organic digestive disorders.

Relationship to Wind

Pain that is associated with burping, flatulence and a sensation of gaseous distension and, in particular, pain that is relieved by the expression of wind, either up or down, is usually non-ulcer rather than ulcer dyspepsia. This generalization should be modified in the case of patients with a peptic ulcer who take a bicarbonate-based antacid. Under those circumstances, the neutralizing action of bicarbonate on gastric acid releases carbon dioxide and so burping often coincides with the relief of pain.

Relationship to Bowel Movement

The pain of colonic disorders often ameliorates temporarily when the bowels move and this is true both with inflammatory (colitis) and motility (irritable bowel) disorders. Although spastic colon pain is usually in the lower abdomen and thus less likely to fall under the heading of dyspepsia, it must be remembered that a substantial proportion, around 30%, of irritable colon sufferers experience their colonic pain in the epigastrium or the hypochondria[9,11,18]. Another characteristic feature of irritable bowel pain is that it is presaged by constipation and that the onset of pain coincides with the change to looser stools[10].

Relationship to Nausea and Vomiting

Peptic ulcer pain, if severe, may cause nausea and vomiting. When this happens the patient will generally feel greatly improved within minutes of vomiting, the pain remits and he can eat again. In an uncomplicated duodenal ulcer, nausea is only an accompaniment of bad pain and does not occur on its own. Nausea, especially on awaking, with mild or absent pain, suggests functional dyspepsia.

Flatulence

Patients vary greatly in what they mean by this. It covers eructation, passage of flatus, borborygmi and a feeling of gaseous distension. Avery Jones[19] has proposed the term 'burbulence' to encompass this spectrum of symptoms. Clearly the normal gut always has a certain amount of gas within it; the stomach contains swallowed air and the colon contains a mixture of swallowed air and gases such as methane, hydrogen and carbon dioxide produced by bacterial fermentation. There is normally relatively little gas within the small intestine. As the expulsion of gastric and colonic gas is a physiological phenomenon, there is no obvious dividing line between normal and abnormal flatulence – more it is in the eye of the beholder. Few gastroenterologists have made gas their research interest, but Levitt, Professor of Medicine at Minnesota, is an exception. He and others have shown that the amount and number of occasions on which flatus is passed each day by normal people is extremely variable and although $\frac{1}{2}$–1 litre is the rule, several litres per day is perfectly healthy. Dietary factors are of prime importance and the amount of colon gas produced by fermentation relates directly to the amount of carbohydrate substrate entering the caecum. Thus it is common knowledge that beans with their high content of poorly digested and absorbed oligosaccharides provide a rich picking for caecal flora and generate much flatus. As a general rule, the amount and quality of flatus passed or wind burped up does not have any pathological correlates. There are one or two minor exceptions – malabsorption leads to particularly foul-smelling flatus because of the fat and protein which gain access to the colonic bacteria, and pyloric stenosis can lead to bacterial fermentation in the sequested gastric contents with ensuing putrid eructation. It must be said though that such circumstances are very uncommon so, by and large, burbulence should be interpreted as a symptom of non-organic dyspepsia. Distension in a more difficult symptom to evaluate and explain. It is one of the most characteristic features of both functional dyspepsia and irritable bowel syndrome. Patients will tell of their difficulty in fastening waistbands and the outward appearance of advanced pregnancy that may change from flat to grossly protuberant in the space of a day. Indeed, many women will be able to demonstrate their abdominal protuberance during the examination. It might be assumed that such patients harbour a large volume of intestinal gas somewhere along the gastrointestinal tract, but such studies as have been done do not show this to be so. Levitt and colleagues[20] infused gas through a tube into the intestines of two groups of subjects and found that for the same volume of infused gas, patients with functional gut disorders suffered much more discomfort and sensations of distension than the normal controls. In functional disorders then, the gut seems over-sensitive to physiological quantities of gas in the gut. The mechanism of the visible distension, particularly that produced at will by women and termed abdominal proptosis, is a change in posture of the spine. By increasing the lumbar lordosis and pushing down the diaphragm, the abdominal contents are forced to the path of least resistance, i.e. forward. This is usually done subconsciously and can be detected by the examining doctor inserting a hand between the couch and the patient's lumbar spine while the distension is being displayed.

Acidity

This is a frequent complaint of dyspeptic patients and open to various interpretations. Some will mean regurgitation of acidic gastric fluid into the mouth with or without associated heartburn. This, I believe, is what most doctors would consider acidity to mean and would be in keeping with a diagnosis of gastro-oesophageal reflux with or without peptic oesophagitis. However, most patients do not give such a description when pressed to define their term. More often the concept is much more vague and consists of a foul taste in the mouth, halitosis or an unpleasant and ill-localized abdominal burning sensation. This sort of acidity is usually functional and if the patient makes much play of the bad taste and foul breath when there is little evidence of poor oral hygiene on examination, it should alert the physician to underlying depression.

Difficulty in Swallowing

Many patients who complain of this as part of their dyspepsia, do not have true dysphagia. True dysphagia should always be assumed to have an organic cause. The patient may complain of difficulty in eating or swallowing when what he actually experiences is globus sensation (a lump in the throat) or early or undue satiety. It may be even less specific than this taking the form of anorexia or nausea for instance.

Nausea and Vomiting

Nausea and vomiting are common, but non-specific associations of a host of organic and non-organic diseases and need careful interpretation. Persistent longstanding nausea, particularly when present on waking, is very suggestive of a functional gastrointestinal problem. Similarly, the complaint of frequent vomiting, especially when a wide variety of foods is held responsible, in the absence of weight loss, is usually non-organic. As mentioned earlier, nausea and vomiting in uncomplicated peptic ulcer is usually an accompaniment to severe pain and the vomiting will afford rapid relief. With functional vomiting, on the other hand, the appetite does not usually reappear and the patient remains nauseated.

Bowel Disturbance

It may not come as second nature to think of bowel disturbance as a part of dyspepsia, but our previously mentioned survey[1] showed that about half of the dyspeptic population included this amongst their symptoms. The predominant pattern in functional dyspepsia is irregular bowel habit with alternating constipation and loose or offensive stools. Careful enquiry will reveal that diarrhoea does not take the form of large volumes of fluid stool, rather the frequent passage of small amounts of unformed stool often with a sense of incomplete evacuation. These symptoms are, of course, typical of an irritable bowel and there is a wide overlap between non-ulcer dyspepsia and the irritable bowel syndrome[10]. This overlap is well-recognized by gastroenterologists, but still seems to baffle clinicians from other fields. It is inherent to the understanding of functional gut disorders that the whole gut is probably irritable or over-sensitive and at different times in a patient's life the symptoms may reflect disorders in a variety of sites.

SPECIFIC SYNDROMES AND AREAS OF MISCONCEPTION

There exist several more or less well-defined clusters of symptoms which are covered by the umbrella of non-ulcer dyspepsia that deserve special mention. I will discuss atypical chest pain and chronic right hypochondrial pain with flatulence.

Atypical Chest Pain

In recent years, there has been an increased recognition that not all anterior chest pain radiating down the left arm is due to ischaemic heart disease and that a sizeable proportion of those admitted to hospital for investigation will turn out to have an alimentary tract disorder. While in some this will be an easily diagnosed organic disease such as peptic oesophagitis, in others the source of the pain is less obvious. There seems good evidence that in some cases there is abnormal oesophageal motility[21]. This is sometimes referred to as the nutcracker oesophagus. Less publicized, but equally well demonstrated, is that the above distribution of pain can occur as a result of colonic motility disorders as in the splenic flexure syndrome described by Dworken[12].

Chronic Right Hypochondrial Pain and Flatulence

By convention this combination of symptoms is thought to indicate gall stones but, as I have already indicated, gall stones cause biliary colic which is quite distinct from chronic right upper quadrant pain, and flatulence is no commoner in those with gall stones than those without. A recent study[11] of 22 patients with this syndrome confirmed the clinical impression that women aged 25–45 are the predominant sufferers, but more usefully demonstrated that the intestine was the organ responsible for the pain. Inflating a balloon within either the small or large intestine or both accurately reproduced the symptoms in 21 of these 22 women. The study also revealed how commonly the symptom complex is over investigated, wrongly diagnosed and inappropriately treated. The patients in question had had their symptoms on average for 9 years, had consulted in all 76 hospital specialists for their complaints, had undergone over 150 imaging investigations of their alimentary tract largely with normal findings and had been subjected to a total of 38 abdominal operations, none of which had cured the pain. It should come as little surprise to know that during a formal, structured interview, half of these patients were found to be depressed. This latter feature is a common attendant of chronic functional abdominal disorders and all too frequently goes undiagnosed[22,23].

Gall Stones and Chronic Cholecystitis

Stones in the gall bladder are common. In the white population of the United Kingdom, Northern Europe and North America, about 10–15% of the adult population harbour stones in the gall bladder and the prevalence increases with age and female sex[14–17]. The prevalence of stones in women of pensionable age is over 30%. From these figures it should be obvious that most gall stones are asymptomatic. In many cases, there is chemical irritation of the gall bladder associated with the stones and in pathological terms this is chronic cholecystitis. The presence of stones floating freely within the gall bladder whether or not there is chronic cholecystitis is not associated with symptoms. Such patients are not immune from flatulent dyspepsia and right upper quadrant discomfort, but these symptoms are equally common in the population without stones or chronic cholecystitis[14–17]. Many textbooks state that Murphy's sign – tenderness over the gall bladder area – is a typical feature of cholelithiasis. This is a most unreliable physical sign which, in fact, has no correlation with uncomplicated gall stones, though it will be present in cases of acute cholecystitis. A positive Murphy's sign is, on the other hand, commonly observed in patients with functional dyspepsia and irritable bowel syndrome and merely emphasizes the over-sensitive nature of the alimentary tract in these conditions. It is difficult to be certain of which organ is actually tender, but in many it is the hepatic flexure of the colon[11]. If a stone becomes impacted in the gall bladder, then symptoms of biliary colic can be expected. The features of biliary colic have already been described in an earlier section. An obstructed cystic duct may also lead to acute cholecystitis or empyema of the gall bladder if the contents of the obstructed bladder become infected. The symptoms of these severe acute inflammatory disorders do not resemble dyspepsia and do not require further elaboration here.

Biliary Dyskinesia[24]

It should now be clear from this review that recurrent right upper quadrant pain with flatulent dyspepsia and fat intolerance does not represent a biliary tract disorder. The terms biliary dyskinesia[25] or dyssynergia[26] have been used particularly in the surgical literature to explain the above symptoms in patients who have been found not to harbour gall stones or any other obvious pathology. These diagnoses should be avoided as they mislead both patient and doctor and inevitably lead to surgery. There are probably occasional cases of true smooth muscle abnormality of the gall bladder or sphincteric region of the common bile duct which give rise to genuine symptoms[24]. Under these circumstances, the symptoms will resemble biliary colic rather than dyspepsia, but the diagnosis should only be made with radiological and biochemical confirmation of an abnormality.

Hiatus Hernia

Hiatus hernia is often used as a clinical diagnosis whereas the term only implies an anatomical feature which may or may not be associated with symptoms. In the past, many have assumed that hiatus hernia is closely associated with oesophageal reflux and peptic oesophagitis. In fact, the correlation between anatomy, physiology and pathology is rather poor[23]. If the symptoms suggest oesophagitis, then this should be the clinical diagnosis. A common problem arises when the patient with typical non-ulcer functional dyspepsia is investigated with barium meal or endoscopy which shows nothing other than hiatus hernia. This probably irrelevant finding is then used to explain the patient's disorder. Treatment with antacids or H_2 blockers is no more successful than placebo and if the patient is unlucky, he is referred for surgery. The results of surgery for hiatus hernia under these circumstances are not good: the anatomy is rearranged, but the symptoms remain.

If the original symptoms are those of oesophagitis and the inflammation can be demonstrated at endoscopy, then surgery has a valuable place. Correction of the hernia with a fundoplication or similar procedure will prevent the reflux and allow the oesophagitis to heal.

GASTRITIS AND DUODENITIS

Gastritis and duodenitis are bona fide pathological terms which indicate mucosal inflammation as assessed by light microscopy. As terms to describe macroscopic mucosal abnormalities demonstrated by barium meal or gastroscopy, they are much less reliable. Used diagnostically to denote a symptomatic clinical disorder, the terms are almost valueless. Balanced and well-referenced reviews of the subject have recently been written by Lagarde and Spiro[28], Joffe and Sankar[29] and Strickland[30].

Gastritis[28,30]

From the purely pathological viewpoint, gastritis is a very common abnormality and has several distinct patterns and a variety of diverse causes. Gastritis has been reported in 50–80% of patients undergoing gastroscopy for all causes including asymptomatic normal subjects. The two main histological types are superficial and atrophic gastritis; the superficial variety may be acute or chronic. There are, in addition, some rare and rather specific forms of gastritis such as chronic erosive gastritis and Ménétrier's giant rugal hypertrophy. The following discussion will be restricted to non-specific chronic gastritis which includes both superficial and atrophic types and accounts for the bulk of the problem.

Superficial gastritis may accompany peptic ulceration, gastric cancer or previous gastric surgery, may be associated with alcohol abuse or treatment with irritant anti-inflammatory drugs or may occur for no evident reason. Atrophic gastritis may be associated with pernicious anaemia, gastric cancer, alcoholism and old age. The differentiation between superficial and atrophic gastritis is not clear cut and there is a gradation of disease between the two poles. Both superficial and atrophic gastritis frequently occur in an asymptomatic population and the incidence increases with age.

Numerous attempts have been made to correlate endoscopic appearances suggesting gastritis (redness, blotchiness and oedema), dyspeptic symptoms and true histological inflammation. It seems that there is no reliable link between these three factors. Certainly some patients with dyspepsia, either ulcer-like or not, will be found to have an angry-looking gastric mucosa endoscopically which on biopsy shows intense inflammation. Unfortunately, it is equally common to find dyspeptic patients without such endoscopic or microscopic appearances and, in addition, asymptomatic subjects who show macroscopic or histological abnormalities. Even the relationship between macroscopic and microscopic gastritis is doubtful because often the intense redness, oedema and blotchiness interpreted as gastritis by the endoscopist is, in fact, simply hyperaemia without any accompanying infiltration with inflammatory cells. It is not so surprising that gastric inflammation is often asymptomatic when one considers Addisonian pernicious anaemia. This condition is invariably associated with marked and longstanding atrophic gastritis histologically, but there are no clinical symptoms to accompany this gastritis.

Duodenitis[28,29]

The picture with duodenitis is really not much clearer than that with gastritis. It is not such a common finding as gastritis. It is nonetheless present in around 30% of patients subjected to gastroscopy for whatever reason. As in the case of gastritis, there is poor correlation between endoscopic assessment of the duodenal mucosa and histological demonstration of inflammation. Similarly, there does not appear to be any constant association between clinical symptoms and inflammation in the duodenum. There are those who believe that duodenitis is part of the duodenal ulcer spectrum, perhaps representing an early phase before the development of macroscopic ulceration. Such believers describe patients with symptoms very suggestive of duodenal ulceration, but in whom only duodenitis has been found; their follow-up studies report that a sizeable proportion of such patients will eventually develop true ulceration. This is not by any means a universal view and others who also believe duodenitis to be a real clinical (as opposed to pathological) entity do not necessarily describe the patients as suffering typical ulcer dyspepsia and deny that the condition has any links with peptic ulceration. Many gastroenterologists, myself included, are still uncertain as to whether duodenitis has any clinical relevance at all in the majority of those who harbour this pathological lesion. Is duodenitis an acid-related disorder? Information on this should help support or contradict an association with duodenal ulcer and might also predict response to treatment. Unfortunately, the evidence available on these points is conflicting with some workers reporting acid hypersecretion in patients with non-ulcer dyspepsia and others showing normal gastric acid output in patients with apparently similar clinical attributes.

What little data there are on the treatment of gastritis and duodenitis serve to suggest that there is no real link between these disorders and peptic ulceration. Antacids and H_2 receptor antagonists produce relief of dyspepsia in some patients with gastroduodenitis, but do not have the same therapeutic benefits as are seen in sufferers of peptic ulceration. The response rate to the drugs in gastroduodenitis is roughly similar to that achieved with placebo and is around 50%[31].

MECHANISMS OF NON-ULCER DYSPEPSIA

There are three proposed mechanisms to explain the symptoms of non-ulcer dyspepsia; they are not necessarily mutually exclusive nor comprehensive. These mechanisms are:

(1) Inflammation

(2) Disordered motility

(3) Psychosomatic.

Inflammation

The first of these (gastroduodenitis) should be straightforward, but as I have already mentioned in the previous section, there is no convincing correlation between symptoms and presence or degree of mucosal inflammation except in a few rather specific instances. A very small proportion of cases with marked endoscopic and histological signs of inflammation do seem to behave similarly to patients with duodenal ulcer both symptomatically and therapeutically. In this small group at least, the inflammation probably causes the symptoms. The same can be said of some patients with chronic erosive gastritis and Menetrier's disease, but even in these more specific pathological disorders, there may be gross macroscopic and microscopic disease in the absence of symptoms. There is also a reasonably persuasive link between dyspeptic symptoms and gastritis caused by alcohol and by certain drugs, e.g. aspirin and non-steroidal anti-inflammatory agents. Sufferers characteristically gain rapid relief of symptoms by abstinence or by stopping the drug and at the same time the endoscopic and histological features of inflammation will resolve.

DISORDERED MOTILITY

The concept of non-ulcer dyspepsia being the result of abnormal motor function of the gut is appealing. Most doctors now accept that the classical irritable bowel syndrome or spastic colon is a colonic motility disorder[10]. It has to be said though that there is not a great deal of reproducible data to confirm that such patients do have a readily recognized pattern of smooth muscle dysfunction. The distal colon is easily accessible to the examining doctor and, at routine sigmoidoscopy, it is common to find that spastic colon sufferers do indeed show visible spasm in the sigmoid and rectum and that distension of the lower bowel with a little air seems to trigger the patient's typical pain. This rather crudely, but satisfactorily, suggests at least that there is an over-activity of smooth muscle contraction and an undue sensitivity to minor degrees of gut distension. The upper gut is, of course, less accessible to routine examination in an unprepared patient. Crude visual assessment of motor activity can be judged by barium cineradiography, but this has several drawbacks. Firstly, it cannot be done by the general practitioner or physician on the spot and requires a third party. Secondly, it is time consuming and expensive and thirdly, it involves a very subjective assessment. There are no clear boundaries between what is normal and what is abnormal in terms of oesophago-gastroduodenal motility provided there is unobstructed passage to the barium column and provided no visceral dilatation is demonstrated.

More objective assessment of upper gut motility can be achieved by manometric studies and by radioisotope techniques. Manometry is unpleasant for the patient as the swallowing of a tube or radiotelemetry capsule is inherent to the technique. Few hospitals have access to manometric equipment and fewer still have clinicians with experience in conducting or interpreting such studies. Radioisotope tests are certainly much more acceptable to the patient and more readily available, but again suffer the problems of interpretation as there are no standardized criteria of normality. For the present, the best that can be said is that a range of putative abnormalities of motility have been reported in non-ulcer dyspepsia: much work in this area has been presented by Professor Johnson's group in Sheffield[32]. Others, in particular Professor Malagelada from the Mayo clinic, have reported a variety of gastric motility disorders in dyspeptic patients. Such disorders cover a spectrum from too little activity (gastric atony)[33] to too much (tachygastria)[34].

Some motility disorders of the oesophagus are readily defined and dyspeptic symptoms from achalasia and scleroderma are well-recognized. As I stated in my earlier definitions, these conditions should not be included in non-ulcer dyspepsia as they have a clearly defined organic basis. The problem with the oesophagus lies in interpreting lesser degrees of abnormality such as tertiary contractions or the rather feeble primary and secondary contractions seen in an elderly population (presbyoesophagus). These disorders are only sometimes associated with symptoms and are commonly encountered in asymptomatic subjects so it is difficult to be sure in the symptomatic individual whether the observed oesophageal activity is cause or coincidence. Overall then, upper gastrointestinal motility disturbance as a cause of non-ulcer dyspepsia is an attractive theory, but remains unproven and unstandardized.

Psychosomatic

There is much evidence from everyday clinical experience to suggest that psychological factors contribute to dyspepsia. We are all familiar with the occasional unpleasant gastrointestinal sensation at times of fear, stress and embarrassment. It seems a logical step to suppose that those with perennial feelings of stress, anxiety states and neuroses may suffer from more chronic alimentary symptoms. There is work to show that patients with functional abdominal symptoms have lower pain thresholds or greater tendencies to report pain than normal subjects[10,23,28]. Psychometric testing indicates that patients with non-ulcer dyspepsia or irritable bowel syndrome are more neurotic and more likely to show features of anxiety, depression and hysteria than other medical patients[22,35]. Not all patients though with functional dyspepsia will have any demonstrable psychological abnormality. The association between life stress and dyspepsia is not straightforward. While some have reported that patients with functional gut symptoms experience more stress than other medical patients prior to hospitalization[23], a very recent study from Australia[36] has shown no such association. As to the mechanism of psychogenic symptoms, one can only speculate. The motility school will suggest that nervous impulses alter gut motility while the neuroendocrine school would consider that nerve endings in the viscera become hypersensitive to normal physiological events with the result that pain is registered at the cortical level without any detectable perturbation in the alimentary tract.

SYMPTOMS OUTSIDE THE GASTROINTESTINAL TRACT IN NON-ULCER DYSPEPSIA

It is common experience that patients with both non-ulcer dyspepsia and irritable bowel syndrome complain of symptoms in other parts of the body more readily than patients with organic gastrointestinal diseases[37]. Under this heading, the most frequent complaints are tiredness, headache, dyspareunia, nocturia, urinary frequency, dysuria, backache, a foul taste in the mouth, dizziness, insomnia and impotence. Many of these symptoms are also features of depression, in particular tiredness, insomnia and impotence. It is also interesting to look at the corollary of this problem. Patients who present to the neurologist with non-organic headaches and patients with urinary symptoms whose urological investigations prove negative, complain of functional dyspeptic and irritable bowel symptoms more commonly than patients with organic causes of headache or those with confirmed urinary tract infections.

Psychiatric Disorders in a Dyspeptic Population

There does not appear to be any relationship between peptic ulcers and psychiatric illness. There is though without doubt such an association in the case of non-ulcer dyspepsia[22,35]. Most often the psychiatric disorder is a minor or trivial disturbance, or indeed just an integral part of the subject's personality. The typical young patient with non-ulcer dyspepsia is the harassed housewife or the aggressive and pressurized businessman who both recognize that their symptoms are directly related to their daily existence. Such patients often say at the initial interview that the symptoms resolve when life is calm, while on holiday or after a few stiff drinks in the evening. This type of history demonstrates psychological influences, suggests a highly strung, sensitive or nervous personality, but cannot be counted as a psychiatric disorder. At the other extreme is the elderly patient presenting with dyspepsia for which no organic cause is evident; he is convinced that he is harbouring sinister pathology, he is tired, lacks all drive and interest, he cannot sleep or concentrate and he cries easily. He is clearly suffering from depression and the dyspepsia is one of the many somatic components of the depressive illness. As in most fields of medicine, the extremes that I have mentioned do not constitute a great proportion of symptomatic patients and, of course, present little in the way of a diagnostic challenge. The majority of patients with non-ulcer dyspepsia will show either no evidence of psychological disturbance or more subtle degrees of anxiety or depression which take a little more detective work. Anxiety is quite commonly expressed by patients and often attributed to the fact that they are suffering abdominal symptoms: it may be difficult to sort out which is the chicken and which the egg. Depression is less readily admitted by patients unless they are specifically pressed on the point: this seems to be a less socially acceptable emotion than anxiety. This is particularly true of endogenous depression where there is no precipitating cause of the depression. Patients feel belittled and guilty that they are depressed without, in their eyes, due reason. This makes them much less inclined to volunteer their emotions and preoccupations spontaneously. It is common too for patients with depression to deny the diagnosis when it is suggested because the somatic features are so strong that they cannot conceive that a 'mental' problem is at the root of the trouble. These are the patients in whom it is essential by skilful history taking to unearth the features of atypical or covert depression because only treatment of this underlying disorder will resolve or at least render acceptable the dyspeptic symptoms. When any painful condition becomes chronic and undiagnosed, whether it is dyspepsia or headache, then accompanying depression is extremely frequent[38]. In most studies where this specific facet has been examined, the prevalence of depression exceeds 50% in patients suffering chronic pain[22,35,38].

INVESTIGATION

In the young patient with a typically non-organic history as already described, particularly when the symptoms are longstanding and there is obvious relation to stress, investigation is unnecessary. It may even be counter-productive by establishing a climate in which the patient is led to believe that the doctor is unsure of his ground and in search of a diagnosis. Sometimes though there is a genuine element of doubt as to whether there is underlying organic disease in which case it is simple enough to explain the differential diagnosis to the patient and to arrange an appropriate test. Most often this will be a barium meal or gastroscopy to confirm or exclude peptic disease. Cholecystography should be avoided in patients with dyspepsia because the information yielded is likely to be irrelevant to the clinical problem. If the cholecystogram is negative, then nothing useful has been gained while if it shows gall stones, then, more often than not, the situation has been complicated rather than simplified. Even though removal of the gall bladder will have an effect no greater than placebo on the patient's dyspepsia, it is very difficult for the doctor to decline to do anything about the gall stones once they have been demonstrated. Unless the presenting symptom is that of biliary colic (see Table 4.2), then the wise physician does not look for trouble – better to let sleeping dogs lie. A similar argument holds for the use of abdominal ultrasound. All too frequently, ultrasound is ordered for patients with vague abdominal symptoms and a chance abnormality such as a small ovarian or renal cyst or gall stones is incorrectly held responsible.

In the older patient with a short history and features to suggest organic disease such as weight loss, then investigation is appropriate and should include full blood count, liver function tests and barium meal or endoscopy. Ultrasound may be indicated depending on the circumstances.

Due warning has already been given in earlier sections about over- or misinterpretation of findings of dubious significance during investigation such as gastritis, duodenitis, hiatus hernia and motility disturbances. Radiologists' comments about the speed or tardiness of gastric emptying or small bowel transit are often misleading. The range of normality is extremely wide and only exceptionally is a very slow or very fast transit time in the absence of any other radiological abnormality a clinically significant finding.

In referral centres with a research interest, it can be helpful to perform special investigations in those patients with intractable symptoms provided the investigations are harmless and produce some benefit for the patient. In selected patients, it can be valuable to try to reproduce the spontaneous abdominal pain by balloon insufflation within the upper or lower gastrointestinal tract[9,11,13]. This can give the patient insight into the over-sensitive nature of his gut and provide an acceptable and comprehensible explanation for his symptoms. I should stress that tests like balloon insufflation are time consuming, require a certain degree of skill for their performance and are non-standardized. I do not recommend they be used except as part of a study programme where sufficient numbers can be done to enable the practitioner to interpret the results.

It is a good rule not to organize complicated, expensive and even dangerous investigations such as CT scan, ERCP, laparoscopy or laparotomy without first having a very shrewd idea that a particular organic disease is likely to be revealed.

TREATMENT

The treatment of non-ulcer dyspepsia is less successful in both the short and long terms than that of peptic ulcer. Unlike the case of peptic ulcer, there is no well accepted efficacious treatment by which to judge the success of others. In a similar vein, while there are many controlled clinical trials of treatment for peptic ulcer, there are precious few for non-ulcer dyspepsia. Treatment can be divided into categories:

(1) Simple symptomatic measures

(2) Dietary or environmental modifications

(3) Antacids

(4) Drugs affecting gut motility

(5) Anti-ulcer drugs

(6) Mood altering drugs

(7) Psychological manoeuvres.

Simple Symptomatic Measures

In many patients with mild dyspepsia, old family remedies seem to settle the symptoms quickly and reliably. Under this heading come simple proprietary medicines and analgesics, especially if effervescent, for instance Andrews, Enos, Alka Seltzer and ordinary soda water. Some of these contain an antacid, though in small quantities. It is interesting that many of the more popular remedies are in fact primarily purgatives and this implies that the link between dyspepsia and irritable bowel is a close one. In our survey of dyspepsia and indigestion[1], we found that almost half of those questioned considered laxatives to be effective in relieving symptoms. Other popular remedies include a hot water bottle or a glass of hot water, aspirin or paracetamol[1].

Dietary and Environmental Modifications

Many sufferers find that avoidance of rich, spicy or fatty food will prevent dyspepsia or lessen its frequency, but there are not to my knowledge any controlled studies to verify this commonly voiced opinion. If the sufferer over indulges in tobacco or alcohol, then abstinence is often an effective cure. Concomitant therapy with aspirin or non-steroidal anti-inflammatory drugs may precipitate dyspepsia and a change in therapy can relieve the situation.

Antacids

Huge quantities of antacids are taken each year by the dyspeptic population, either bought across the counter or prescribed by a doctor[28,39,40]. This should imply that they are of great value, but when the literature on the subject is carefully reviewed, then there is no convincing evidence to show that antacids have any particular benefit in non-ulcer dyspepsia. The few studies which report to show beneficial effect were so badly designed that conclusions could not justly be drawn[28]. In the better controlled studies, the effect of antacids was equal to placebo[2,28,31]. Certain additives to standard magnesium or aluminium based antacids may or may not have a therapeutic effect. The peppermint flavouring possibly has an effect, though in the doses added, this is more likely by suggestion than by pharmacology. Dimethicone is meant to reduce flatulence, but controlled studies do not confirm this. Bicarbonate will effervesce and the resultant burping will make many patients feel better[1].

Drugs affecting Gut Motility

Anti-spasmodics and anti-cholinergics have been in use for many years and in some patients seem to work well. Propantheline, encapsulated peppermint oil and mebeverine have their devotees, but it is difficult to find well-conducted studies to prove their value. Drugs to increase gastric motility such as metaclopropamide and domperidone[28] have paradoxically also been used with some success in non-ulcer dyspepsia, but again there is little controlled data to verify their worth.

Anti-ulcer Drugs

As there is no convincing link between ulcer and non-ulcer dyspepsia except perhaps in a few patients with severe duodenitis, then one would not anticipate that drugs which heal ulcers would have any therapeutic action in non-ulcer dyspepsia. This, of course, has not prevented enthusiastic drug companies from promoting the use of their expensive anti-ulcer drugs in patients without ulcers nor has it prevented uncritical doctors prescribing them. Claims have been made for the efficacy of H_2 receptor antagonists cimetidine and ranitidine[28,41] and of pirenzepine[42], but the evidence is not convincing and other trials have shown that the success of these drugs is similar to that achieved with placebo[31,43].

Mood Altering Drugs

In patients with stress induced dyspepsia, there is sometimes a marked improvement with an anxiolytic drug. Such drugs are only of value when used for short periods as they both lose their anxiolytic properties and induce dependence when used for more than a few weeks. In patients with chronic dyspepsia and chronic anxiety, their use is to be discouraged as it will not produce any lasting benefit and may lead to worse problems than those for which treatment was originally given.

As I have pointed out in an earlier section, depression is frequently associated with functional abdominal symptoms, particularly when these symptoms are reported by the patient as severe enough to dominate their entire outlook. Treatment of dyspepsia under these circumstances is usually quite fruitless unless the depression itself is treated first. More often than not, once the depression has lifted, it is actually no longer necessary to give treatment for the dyspepsia as the patient can contend with the now mild symptoms using the simple measures available to the general dyspeptic population.

Psychological Manoeuvres

The simplest and often the most effective management of stress related dyspepsia is explanation and discussion with the sufferer. The underlying worries of the patient may not at first be obvious, but a receptive and understanding doctor may find out for instance that someone close to the patient has recently had diagnosed or died from a gastric cancer. Strong reassurance after taking a detailed history and performing a thorough examination is worth infinitely more than a request for a barium meal and a prescription for the pharmaceutical flavour of the month.

At a more sophisticated level or in cases where there is a greater degree of psychological or psychiatric upset, then there is possibly a place for a more formal approach. Both psychotherapy and hypnotherapy have been used for patients with functional gut disorders with variable response rates. A recent trial of hypnotherapy in irritable bowel syndrome produced remarkable results[44], but the study came in for some criticism and has not, so far, been confirmed by other workers. Such an approach is probably only applicable to a very small minority of patients with intractable symptoms because it is so time consuming.

Overview of Treatment

From the foregoing, it is apparent that there is no well-proven effective treatment, though many remedies seem to afford adequate relief. It is sensible to take a pragmatic approach. Start with reassurance and treatment of any underlying psychiatric disorder, particularly depression, and make sure that the patient is not responsible for inducing his symptoms with tobacco, alcohol or irritant drugs. If this fails, then try antacids, antacid aperient combinations, anti-spasmodics or a drug to stimulate gastric emptying. I can find no justification for using specific anti-ulcer drugs. It is important for the patient to be made to realize that quite often no drug or regime will have any useful effect and that he will have to learn to live with the complaint in the knowledge that it will do no harm.

REFERENCES

1. Kingham, J. G. C., Fairclough, P. D. and Dawson, A. M. (1983). What is indigestion? *J. R. Soc. Med.*, **76**, 183–186
2. Knill Jones, R. P. (1985). A formal approach to symptoms in dyspepsia. *Clin. Gastroenterol.*, **14**, 517–529
3. Harvey, R. F., Silih, S. Y. and Read, A. E. (1983). Organic and functional disorders in 2000 gastroenterology outpatients. *Lancet*, **1**, 632–634
4. Thompson, W. G. and Heaton, K. W. (1980). Functional bowel disorder in apparently healthy people. *Gastroenterology*, **79**, 283–288
5. Moynihan, B. G. A. (1905). On duodenal ulcer with notes of 52 operations. *Lancet*, **1**, 340–346
6. Horrocks, J. C. and De Dombal, F. T. (1978). Clinical presentation of patients with dyspepsia. *Gut*, **19**, 19–26
7. Crean, G. P. (1985). Towards a positive diagnosis of irritable bowel

syndrome. In Read, N. W. (ed.) *Irritable Bowel Syndrome*, pp. 29–42, (London: Grune and Stratton)

8. Horrocks, J. C. and De Dombal, F. T. (1975). Diagnosis of dyspepsia from data collected by a physician's assistant. *Br. Med. J.*, **3**, 421–423

9. Swarbrick, E. T., Hegarty, J. E., Bat, L., Williams, C. B. and Dawson, A. M. (1980). Site of pain from the irritable bowel. *Lancet*, **2**, 443–446

10. Thompson, W. G. (1979). *The Irritable Gut*, p. 18. (Baltimore: University Park Press)

11. Kingham, J. G. C. and Dawson, A. M. (1985). Origin of chronic right upper quadrant pain. *Gut*, **26**, 783–788

12. Dworken, H. J. (1952). Supradiaphragmatic reference of pain from the colon. *Gastroenterology*, **22**, 222–231

13. Moriarty, K. J. and Dawson, A. M. (1982). Functional abdominal pain – further evidence that whole gut is affected. *Br. Med. J.*, **284**, 1670–1672

14. Hinkel, C. L. and Moller, G. A. (1957). Correlation of symptoms, age, sex and habits with cholecystographic findings in 1000 consecutive examinations. *Gastroenterology*, **32**, 807–815

15. Koch, J. P. and Donaldson, R. M. (1964). A survey of food intolerances in hospitalized patients. *N. Engl. J. Med.*, **271**, 13, 657–660

16. Bainton, D. (1976). Gall bladder disease. *N. Engl. J. Med.*, **294**, 1147–1149

17. Price, W. H. (1963). Gall bladder dyspepsia. *Br. Med. J.*, **3**, 138–141

18. Waller, S. L. and Misiewicz, J. J. (1969). Prognosis in the irritable bowel syndrome. *Lancet*, **2**, 753–756

19. Jones, A. F. (1967). Burbulence. *Practitioner*, **198**, 367–370

20. Lasser, R. B., Bond, J. H. and Levitt, M. D. (1975). The role of intestinal gas in functional abdominal pain. *N. Engl. J. Med.*, **293**, 524–626

21. Benjamin, S. B., Gerhardt, D. C. and Castell, D. O. (1979). High amplitude, peristaltic oesophageal contractions associated with chest pain and/or dysphagia. *Gastroenterology*, **77**, 478–483

22. Gomez, Joan and Dally, P. (1977). Psychologically mediated abdominal pain in surgical and medical outpatient clinics. *Br. Med. J.*, **1**, 1451–1453

23. Thompson, W. G. (1984). Non-ulcer dyspepsia. *Can. Med. Assoc. J.*, **1**, 330, 565–569

24. Carr-Locke, D. L. (1984). Biliary dyskinesia, gall bladder dyskinesia and biliary stenosis. In Bouchier, I. A. D., Allan, R. N., Hodgson, H. J. F. and Keighley, M. R. C. (eds.) *Textbook of Gastroenterology*, pp. 1428–1450 (London: Balliere Tindall)

25. Ivy, A. C. (1934). Biliary dyskinesia. *Ann. Intern. Med.*, **8**, 115–122

26. Best, R. R. and Hicken, N. F. (1936). Cholangiographic demonstration of biliary dyssynergia. *J. Am. Med. Assoc.*, **107**, 1615–1620

27. Pope, C. E. (1976). Pathophysiology and diagnosis of reflux oesophagitis. *Gastroenterology*, **70**, 445–454

28. Lagarde, S. P. and Spiro, H. M. (1984). Non-ulcer dyspepsia. *Clin. Gastroenterol.*, **13**, 437–446

29. Joffe, S. N. and Sankar, M. Y. (1984). Duodenitis. In Bouchier, I. A. D.,

Allan, R. N., Hodgson, H. J. F. and Keighley, M. R. B. (eds.) *Textbook of Gastroenterology*, pp. 125–128 (London: Balliere Tindall)
30. Strickland, R. G. (1984). Gastritis. In Bouchier, I. A. D., Allan, R. N., Hodgson, H. J. F. and Keighley, M. R. B. (eds.) *Textbook of Gastroenterology*, pp. 113–124. (London: Balliere Tindall)
31. Nyron, O., Adami, H., Bates, S., Bergstrom, R., Gustavsson, S., Loof, L. and Nyberg, A. (1986). Absence of therapeutic benefit from antacids or Cimetidine in non-ulcer dyspepsia. *N. Engl. J. Med.*, **314**, 339–343
32. Johnson, A. G. (1975). Cholecystectomy and gall stone dyspepsia. *Ann. R. Coll. Surg. Engl.*, **56**, 69–80
33. Stanghellini, V. and Malagelada, J. (1983). Gastric manometric abnormalities in patients with dyspeptic symptoms after fundoplication. *Gut*, **24**, 790–797
34. You, C. H., Lee, K. Y., Chey, W. Y. and Menguy, R. (1980). Electrographic study of patients with unexplained nausea, bloating and vomiting. *Gastroenterology*, **79**, 311–314
35. Hill, O. W. and Blendis, L. (1967). Physical and psychological evaluation of non-organic abdominal pain. *Gut*, **8**, 221–229
36. Talley, N. J. and Piper, D. W. (1986). Major life event stress and dyspepsia of unknown cause: a case controlled study. *Gut*, **27**, 127–134
37. Whorwell, P. J., McCallum, M., Creed, F. H. and Roberts, C. T. (1986). Non-colonic features of irritable bowel syndrome. *Gut*, **27**, 37–40
38. Kramlinger, K. G., Swanson, D. W. and Maruta, T. (1983). Are patients with chronic pain depressed? *Am. J. Psychiatry*, **140**, 747–749
39. Petersen, H. (1981). Further investigations and treatment of non-ulcer dyspepsia. *Scand. J. Gastroenterol.*, **17** (Suppl. 79), 130–134
40. Tyllstrom, J., Adami, H., Agenas, I., Gustavsson, S., Loof, L., Nyberg, A., Nyren, O. and Wilholm, B. (1984). The clinical diagnosis of gastritis – aspects of current therapy and drug consumption. *Scand. J. Gastroenterol.*, **19**, 755–760
41. Saunders, J. H. B., Oliver, R. J. and Higson, D. L. (1986). Dyspepsia: incidence of non-ulcer disease in a controlled trial of Ranitidine in general practice. *Br. Med. J.*, **292**, 665–668
42. Giorgi-Conciato, M., Daniotti, S. and Ferrarri, P. A. *et al.* (1982). Efficacy and safety of Pirenzepine in peptic ulcer and in non-ulcerous gastroduodenal diseases. A multicentre controlled clinical trial. *Scand. J. Gastroenterol.*, **17** (Suppl. 81), 1–41
43. Lance, P., Filipe, M. I., Schiller, K. F. R. and Wastell, C. (1981). Cimetidine for non-ulcer dyspepsia. *Gastroenterology*, **80**, 1203
44. Whorwell, P. J., Prior, A. and Faragher, E. B. (1984). Controlled trial of hypnotherapy in the treatment of severe refractory irritable bowel syndrome. *Lancet*, **2**, 1232–1233

INDEX